Rhythm Quizlets - II

by

Henry J.L. Marriott, M.D

CBR Publishing Corporation

Second Edition

CBR Publishing Corporation
1001 Wall Street
El Paso, Texas 79915
800-544-3324

FOREWORD

This collection of arrhythmias embraces both the simple and the sophisticated—from the simple extrasystole and the basic A-V Wenckebach to concealed conduction and the sophisticated tachyarrhythmia. Though not methodically arranged in order of complexity, the simpler tracings are all in the early part of the book with the more complex ones in the latter half.

Because ladder diagrams play such an important role in unravelling some of the more difficult arrhythmias, "ladders" are printed under most of the tracings to encourage practice and proficiency in using them. Many a tracing fails to yield up its secret until its message is translated into the language of the ladder; conversely, many a hasty assumption experiences rejection upon exposure to the ladder's constraints. I therefore strongly recommend cultivating a familiarity with their use.

The tracings are printed on the left hand page prefaced by a brief description of the patient—because it is important to treat, not just the arrhythmia, but the-patient-with-the- arrhythmia; answers are opposite on the right hand page. In each case, ask (and answer!) two questions:

What is the arrhythmic diagnosis?

What is an appropriate therapy FOR THIS PATIENT?

Cover the right hand page while you're working on the left.

Henry J. L. Marriott, M.D.

ABBREVIATIONS: NOTICE TO READER

The following abbreviations are in such general use that they will be used in this text without further notice:

A-V -	atrioventricular
BBB -	bundle-branch block
CCU -	coronary care unit
I-V -	intravenous
LBBB -	left bundle-branch block
min -	minute
RBBB -	right bundle-branch block
s -	second
VPB -	ventricular premature beat (extrasystole)

TABLE OF CONTENTS

1. From a 46-year old white woman with pulmonary emphysema and cor pulmonale.

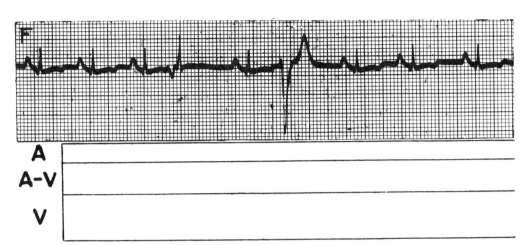

#1

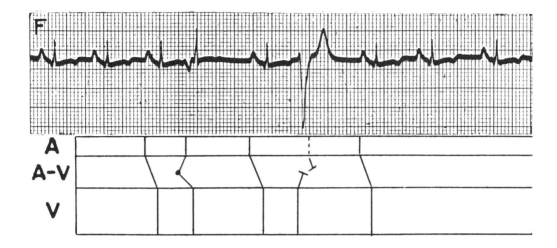

DIAGNOSIS: Sinus rhythm (rate 100/min), interrupted by one supraventricular (probably junctional) and one ventricular premature beat.

SPECIAL POINTS: The occurence of both ventricular and supraventricular extrasystoles in the same tracing is thought to be good evidence of myocardial disease. In this case, of course, there are also obvious T wave abnormalities in this lead (aVF) and the peaked P waves of cor pulmonale.

The supraventricular premature beat could be ectopic atrial or junctional; because of the short P′-R interval (less than 0.12 s) most authorities would favor junctional (see laddergram).

TREATMENT: The vast majority of extrasystoles should not be treated — and that certainly applies to these unless they become symptomatically troublesome.

2. From a 56-year old man with classical angina of effort; receiving nifedipine and nitroglycerine p.r.n.

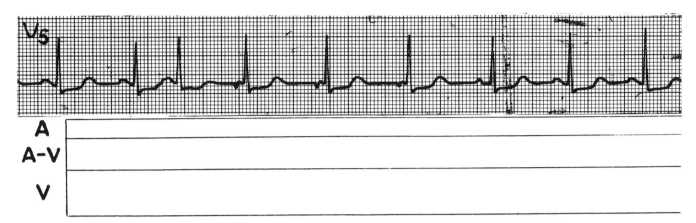

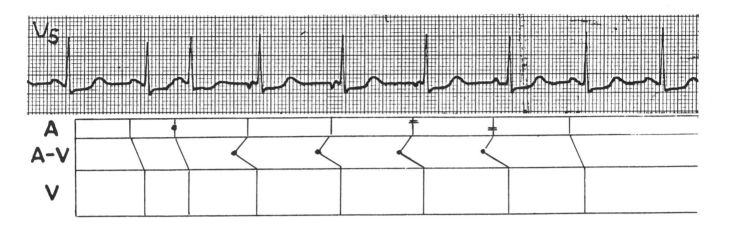

DIAGNOSIS: Sinus rhythm interrupted by an atrial premature beat which initiates a shift of pacemaker to an accelerated junctional rhyghm. After two retrograde P waves, the following two P waves almost certainly represent atrial fusion between sinus and retrograde impulses (see laddergram). The last beats are sinus beats.

TREATMENT: None required

3. From a 3-month old infant with terminal febrile illness; autopsy revealed abscesses in the myocardium.

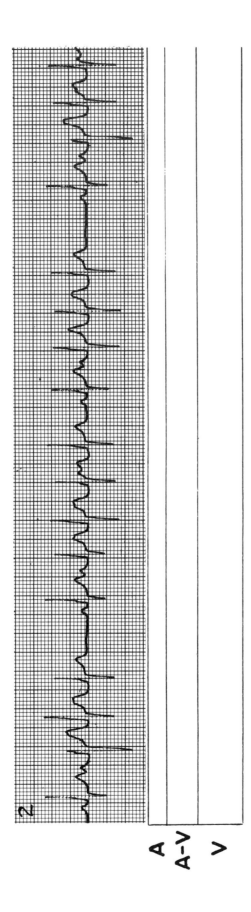

#3 DIAGNOSES: Short bursts of irregular atrial tachycardia. Left anterior hemiblock aberration in two of the beats.

SPECIAL POINT: Aberration, of course, is most likely to develop in the second beat in a run of rapid beats because, by definition, this is the only beat that ends a short cycle preceded by a relatively long one; and the longer cycle lengthens the ensuing refractory period, setting the stage for aberration, especially if the next beat is early.

TREATMENT: Ectopic atrial activity is often a sign of congestive heart failure and if there is any suspicion of this, a digitalis preparation is the drug of choice. For a general approach to the treatment of supraventricular tachycardias, see page 109.

4. From a 67-year old man with fever, uremia, pericardial rub and blood pressure of 200/112.

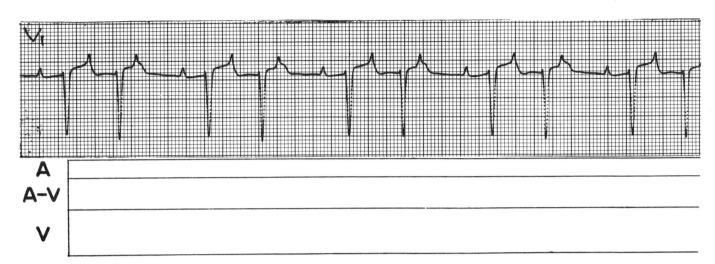

A

A-V

V

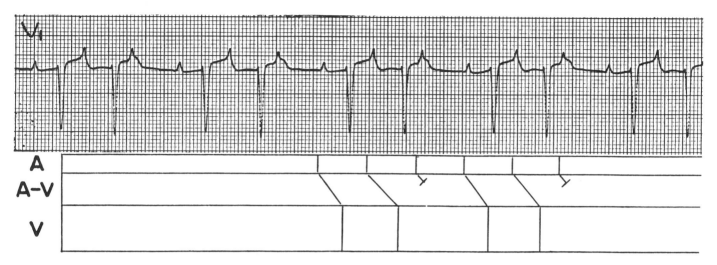

DIAGNOSIS: Sinus or ectopic atrial tachycardia (rate 116/min) with 3:2 A-V Wenckebach periods.

SPECIAL POINTS: 3:2 Wenckebach conduction is a common cause of bigeminal rhythm. The origin of P waves shaped like these is uncertain: Retrograde P waves in V1 are often sharply pointed and positive, but there is no way to exclude a sinus or ectopic atrial mechanism.

TREATMENT: The tachycardia is probably sinus and will abate with resolution of his febrile state. For a general approach to the treatment of supraventricular tachycardias, see page 109. The type I A-V block requires no treatment; for a general approach to the treatment of A-V block, see page 113.

5. From a 63-year old hypertensive black woman (BP 190/118); she had left ventricular enlargement on physical examination but no symptoms and was taking no medications.

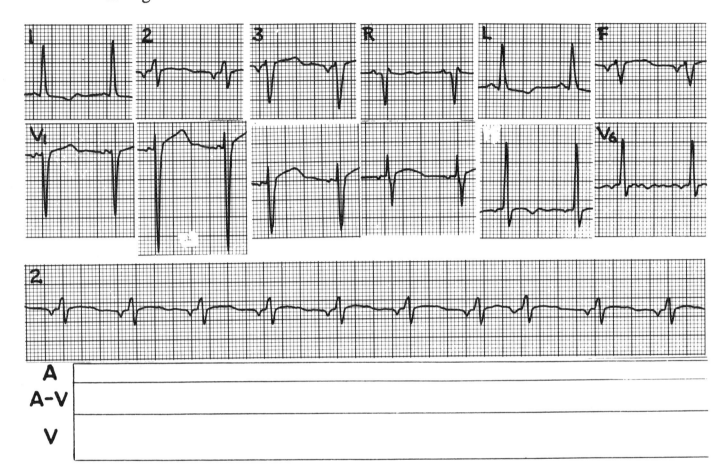

#5 DIAGNOSIS: Accelerated junctional rhythm, rate 76/min; in the rhythm strip of lead 2, the regular junctional rhythm is interrupted by one atrial premature beat. The left axis deviation (-30°) may be due to delay in the anterior fascicle; and the rather high voltage (leads 1, V2 and V5) and ST-T pattern suggest left ventricular enlargement.

SPECIAL POINT: Note the typical polarity of retrograde P waves: Inverted leads 2, 3 and aVF, upright in 1, aVR and aVL, diphasic (-+) in V1 (in contrast with the diphasic sinus P wave which is usually +-), and inverted in V5 and V6.

TREATMENT: Leave the rhythm alone—but treat the hypertension!

6. From an asymptomatic 8-year old boy. (The strips are continuous).

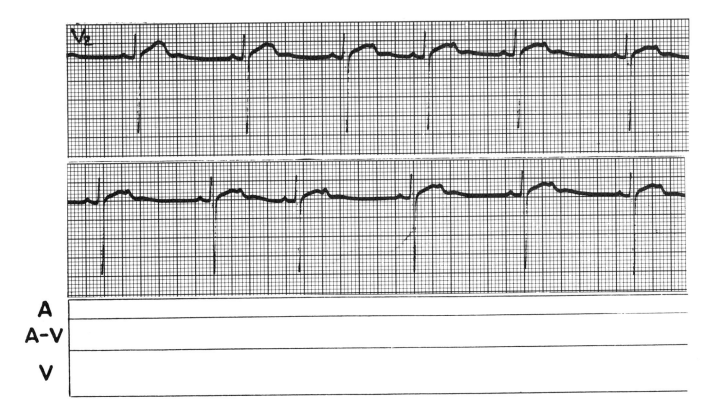

A

A-V

V

#6 **DIAGNOSIS:** Sinus bradycardia with arrhythmia (in a child).

SPECIAL POINT: Bifid T waves, like these, are a pediatric trap— the second bump is often mistaken for a P wave. The clue, as in this case, is that the P-like wave is constantly related to the preceding QRS and is out of step with the evident sinus P waves.

Treatment: Obviously none.

7. From a 51-year old hypertensive black man (BP 184/116) with frequent palpitations.

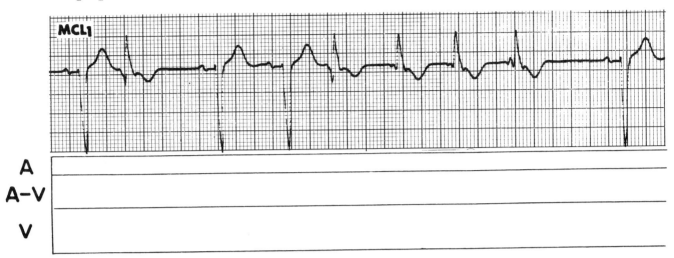

A

A–V

V

#7 DIAGNOSIS: After one sinus beat, there is an isolated left ventricular extrasystole. Two returning sinus beats are followed by a run of accelerated idioventricular rhythm (AIVR) presumably from the same ectopic focus.

SPECIAL POINTS: It is not uncommon for an ectopic ventricular focus to spawn more then one manifestation of ectopic rhythm.

The Q wave and T wave inversion in the isolated VPB and in the one that initiates the AIVR suggest the probability of an associated, probably old, anterior infarction.

TREATMENT: Whether ventricular extrasystoles should be treated or not depends entirely on the clinical context (see general approach on page 106). AIVR almost never requires therapy.

8. From a 72-year old man with a history of myocardial infarction six years earlier. He has since done quite well, but for the past week has felt an unaccustomed weakness and the awareness of intermittent pulsations in his neck. (The strips are continuous).

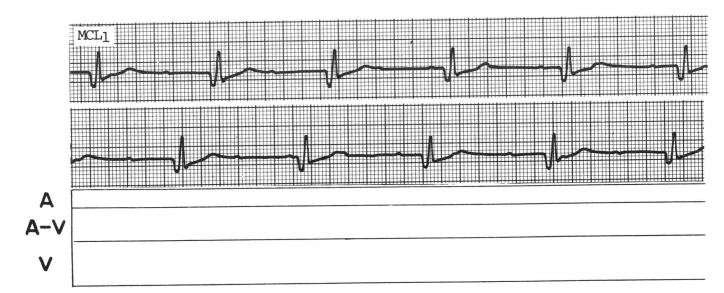

#8 DIAGNOSIS: Probable complete A-V block with idioventricular escape rhythm (rate 47/min).

SPECIAL POINTS: Because the ventricular rate does not quite reach the requirement of being "slow enough," i.e., under 45/min, this should be labelled only <u>probable</u> complete A-V block.

The wide Q waves—even in an ectopic ventricular rhythm—are evidence of the old anterior infarction.

TREATMENT: Since there is no acute cause, the block is probably related to the underlying ischemic disease; the patient is significantly symptomatic and therefore will require a permanent pacemaker.

9. From a 86-year old man with acute inferior myocardial infarction two days ago. Now asymptomatic except for awareness of irregular heart beat.

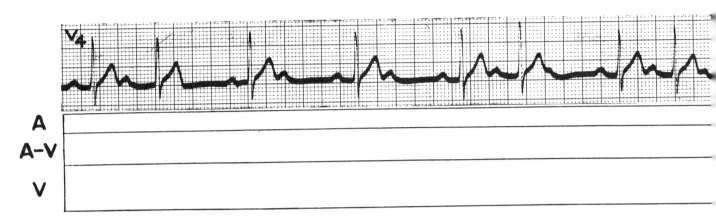

A

A-V

V

#9 DIAGNOSIS: Type I A-V block with 2:1 and 3:2 conduction.

SPECIAL POINTS: During the 2:1 conduction, note the combination of prolonged P-R with normal QRS—the typical secondary features of type I block. (Compare and contrast these findings with those in type II block, see #11).

TREATMENT: None at present. For a general approach to the treatment of A-V block, see page 113.

10. From a 47-year old white man with retrosternal pain on exertion; receiving nitroglycerine and diltiazem.

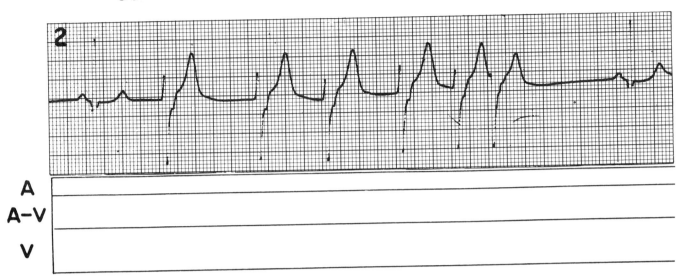

A

A-V

V

#10 **DIAGNOSIS:** A six-beat, self-terminating, run of ectopic ventricular rhythm beginning at a rate of 60/min and accelerating to a rate of 160/min.

SPECIAL POINT: There is no special term for this phenomenon, but it is not uncommon to see bursts of ectopic beats that run the gamut of cycles that represent idioventricular rhythm, accelerated rhythm and tachycardia.

TREATMENT: The rapid acceleration manifested clearly demonstrates the potential for developing ventricular tachycardia; the patient should be treated with a view to preventing sustained ventricular tachycardia. Empirically, propranolol might prove successful. For a general approach to the treatment of ventricular tachycardia, see page 108.

11. From an 86-year old woman, previously healthy, who developed weakness and dizziness yesterday. She reported to the Emergency Room and this tracing was recorded.

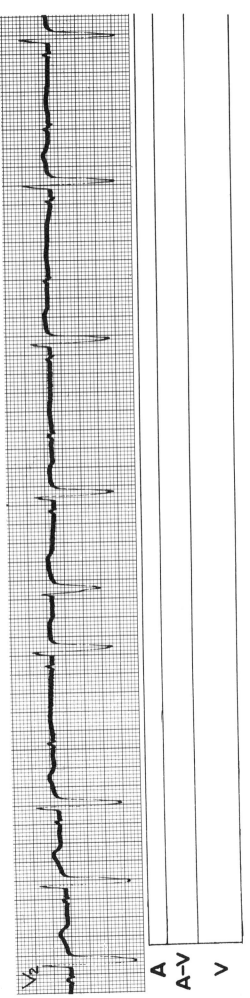

V₂

A

A–V

V

22

#11 **DIAGNOSIS:** Sinus rhythm with type II A-V block, including a run of 2:1 conduction interrupted by one right ventricular extrasystole; LBBB.

SPECIAL POINT: Note the secondary characteristics of type II block: Normal P-R and BBB.

TREATMENT: Genuine type II block—which this clearly is—requires implantation of a permanent pacemaker.

12. From a 5-year old boy one month after surgery for an atrial septal defect.

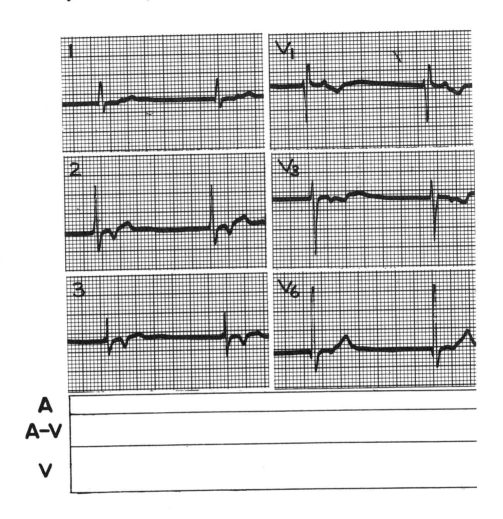

#12 **DIAGNOSIS:** Sick sinus with junctional escape rhythm (rate 45/min) and retrograde conduction (P′ waves following QRS at R-P interval of 0.18 s).

SPECIAL POINTS: For the junction to be in control at this rate, there must be an ailing sinus node (probably injured during surgery)—and this is the primary diagnosis. Note the characteristic polarity of retrograde P waves: Inverted in 2, 3 and V6; partially upright in lead 1 and sharp and upright in V1.

TREATMENT: This is usually a stable rhythm and no treatment is required—beyond prayer for recovery of the sinus node. For a general approach to the treatment of sick sinus syndromes, see page 112.

13. From a 48-year old man complaining of palpitations, but no other symptoms.

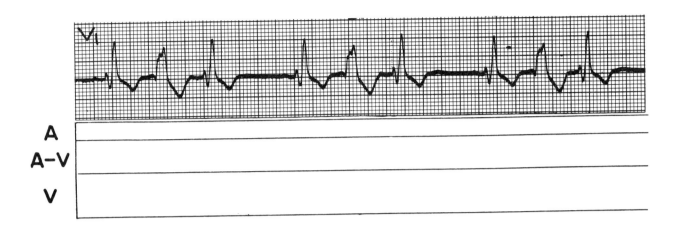

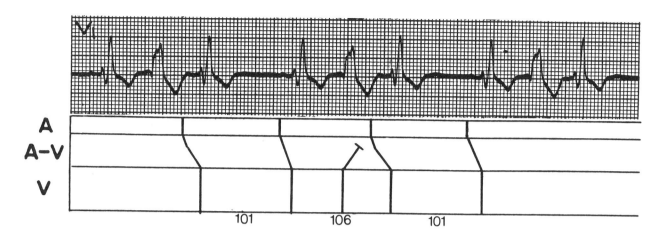

DIAGNOSIS: Sinus bradycardia (rate 58/min) with RBBB and interpolated left ventricular extrasystoles every third best producing trigeminal grouping.

SPECIAL POINT: The sinus cycle containing the interpolated ectopic beat is slightly but measurably longer (1.06 s) than the undisturbed sinus cycles (1.01 s)—see laddergram. This is evidence that there was (concealed) retrograde conduction from the ectopic beat slightly prolonging the subsequent P-R.

TREATMENT: For a general approach to the treatment of ventricular extrasystoles, see page 106.

14. From a 45-year old woman with hypertrophic cardiomyopathy complaining of palpitations.

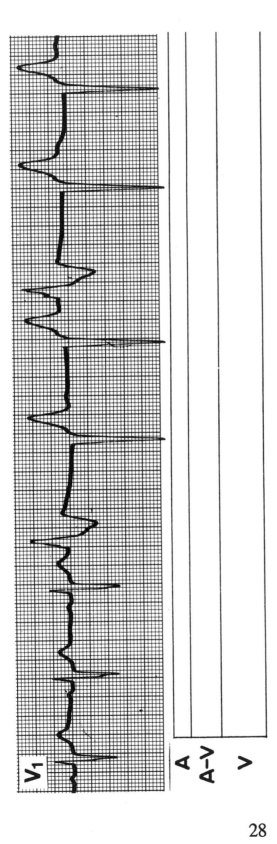

V₁

A

A–V

V

#14

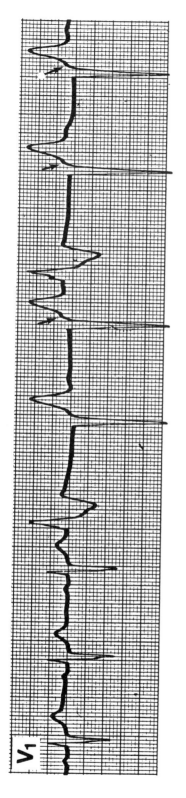

V₁

DIAGNOSIS: After three sinus beats, a left ventricular extrasystole provides a long enough postectopic cycle for an accelerated right ventricular rhythm to escape at rate 58/min; the escaping rhythm captures the atria (retrograde conduction— arrows), and is interrupted by another extrasystole. Although their P waves are not identifiable, measurement indicates that there must also have been retrograde conduction from the ventricular extrasystoles.

SPECIAL POINT: It is always important to distinguish between failure of conduction because of A-V block and failure because of lack of opportunity for A-V conduction. Here there is no evidence of A-V block.

TREATMENT: Escape rhythms should never be treated—they are rescuing rhythms; but in this case the escaping mechanism is mildly accelerated and the V-A sequence of activation resulting from retrograde conduction is depriving the individual of his normal atrial transport function. If this is hemodynamically embarrassing (as it might be in the context of an acute myocardial infarction), it might prove necessary to accelerate the sinus rate with atropine in order to recapture the ventricles and restore the atrial kick.

29

15. From a 41-year old woman, taking "the pill" and with evidence of repeated small pulmonary emboli. (The strips are not continuous).

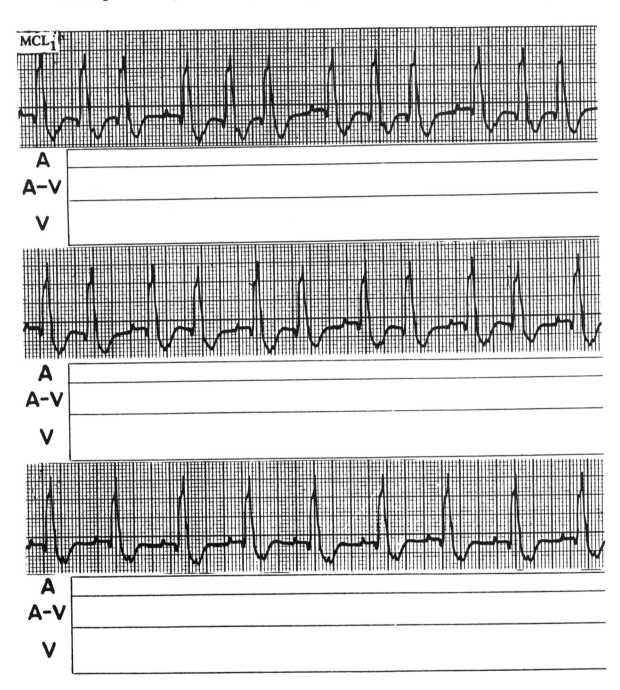

#15 DIAGNOSIS: Atrial tachycardia with rate-dependent A-V conduction ratios: top strip - atrial rate 148/min with 4:3 Wenckebachs; middle strip - atrial rate 152 with 3:2 Wenckebachs; bottom strip - atrial rate 162 with 2:1 conduction.

SPECIAL POINT: Always remember that the pattern of A-V conduction may depend as much on the atrial rate as on the conduction capability of the A-V node.

TREATMENT: For a general approach to the treatment of supraventricular tachyarrhythmias, see page 109.

16. From a 69-year old woman with longstanding history of mitral stenosis and repeated attacks of tachycardia; taking oral verapamil.

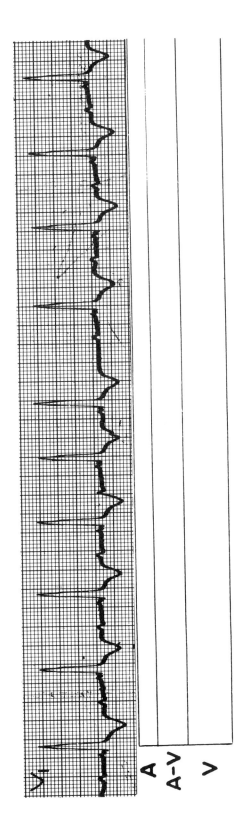

A

A–V

V

#16 **DIAGNOSIS:** Sinus rhythm with first degree A-V block (P-R = 0.26 s) and RBBB interrupted by two atrial premature beats (APBs)

SPECIAL POINTS: The important caveat is not to mistake the initial r of the RBBB pattern for an extra P wave—this error would lead to the diagnosis of a non-existent atrial tachycardia.

Note that the two APBs produce mild overdrive suppression of the sinus rhythm (longer returning cycles).

TREATMENT: None, unless there is some special reason for eliminating the APBs (see discussion on page 107).

17. From a 70-year old man with recent anterior myocardial infarction, a blood pressure of 90/60 and this tachycardia.

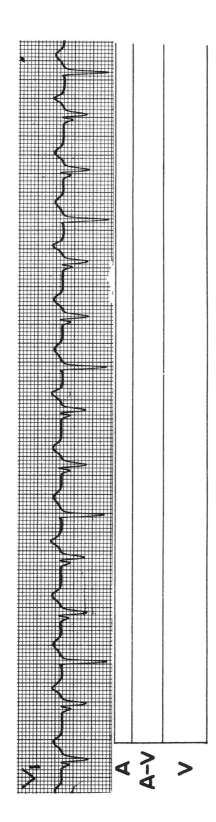

#17

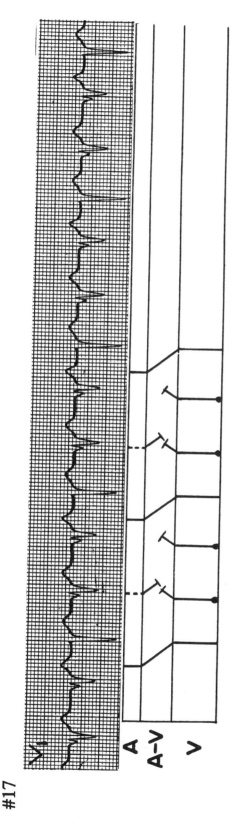

DIAGNOSIS: Ventricular tachycardia (rate 102/min) with resulting A-V dissociation and every third beat a ventricular capture with prolonged P-R interval (see laddergram).

SPECIAL POINTS: The P waves of the conducted sinus beats conspicuously peak the T waves of every third beat (alternate P waves are lost within the ectopic ventricular complex).

TREATMENT: The ventricular tachycardia, though not very fast, in this clinical context should be terminated promptly before further hemodynamic deterioration occurs. For a general approach to the treatment of ventricular tachycardia, see page 108.

35

18. From a 78-year old white man admitted to CCU with severe retrosternal pain; this rhythm strip was recorded on admission, when his blood pressure was 110/68.

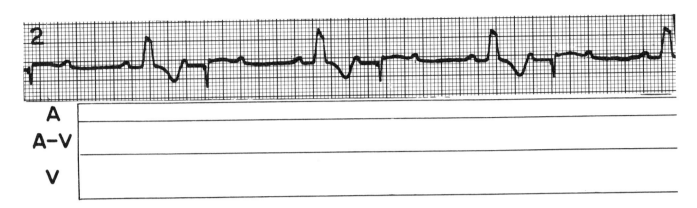

A

A–V

V

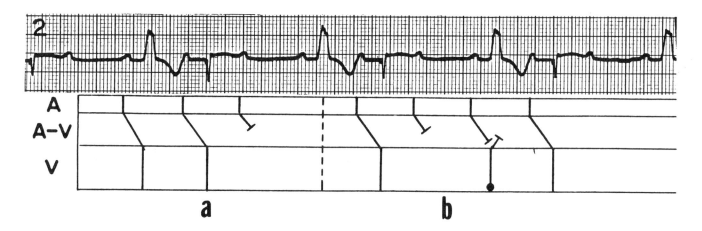

DIAGNOSIS: Inferior infarction with two main possibilities: 2:1 type I A-V block with resulting ventricular escape producing a form of escape-capture bigeminy (laddergram 'b'); or it may be a 3:2 A-V Wenckebach with the wide QRS representing a conducted sinus beat with paradoxical critical rate LBBB (laddergram 'a').

TREATMENT: Type I A-V block in inferior infarction seldom requires active therapy—and this patient's average ventricular rate is adequate at 62/min. For a general approach to the treatment of A-V block, see page 113.

19. From a 50-year old woman who developed severe retrosternal pain 12 hours before these rhythm strips were taken in CCU. In the 15-minute interval between upper and lower strips, the patient in the next room "coded."

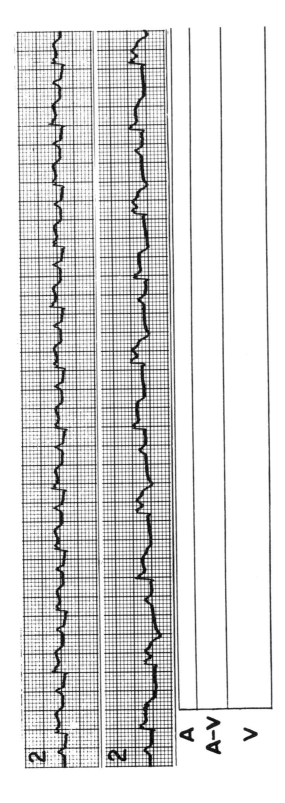

A

A–V

V

#19 DIAGNOSIS: <u>Top strip</u>: sinus rhythm with mild first degree A-V block (P-R = 0.23 s). <u>Bottom strip:</u> type I A-V block with 3:2 Wenckebach periods.

SPECIAL POINT: This illustrates the paramount importance of atrial rate in determining the A-V conduction pattern (compare #15). At an atrial rate of 94, this patient conducts 1:1 with mild P-R prolongation. But with an atrial rate of 112—precipitated by the alarm engendered by the neighboring "code"— so-called "second degree" A-V block develops with 3:2 Wenckebach periods.

TREATMENT: Type I A-V block is a common complication of acute inferior infarction and almost never requires therapy, provided the ventricular rate remains adequate (compare #18, and for general approach to the treatment of A-V block, see page 113).

20. From a 44-year old black man with a dilated cardiomyopathy, massive cardiomegaly, and frank congestive heart failure; receiving diuretics, no digitalis.

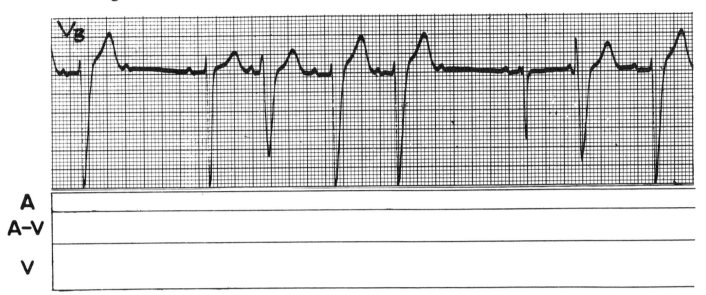

#20 **DIAGNOSIS:** Sinus rhythm with type II A-V block and rate-dependent LBBB; two ventricular extrasystoles.

SPECIAL POINTS: The block is type II because the beats are dropped after consecutive beats have been conducted with the same P-R interval (0.20 s); the normal P-R and a BBB are also typical features of type II block. Rate dependence of the BBB is recognized by the fact that intraventricular conduction improves at the end of the longer cycles. The ventricular extrasystoles are precipitated by lengthened preceding cycles, thus obeying the "rule of bigeminy."

TREATMENT: Genuine type II A-V block (as this probably is) is an unequivocal indication for a permanent artificial pacemaker. For a general approach to treatment of A-V block, see page 113.

21. From a 54-year old white man who suffered an acute inferior infarction two days before this rhythm strip was recorded; his blood pressure at the time of this tracing was 88/68.

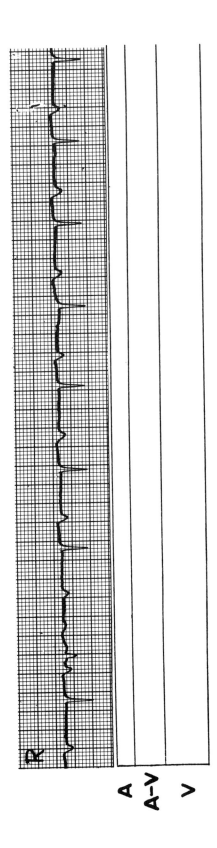

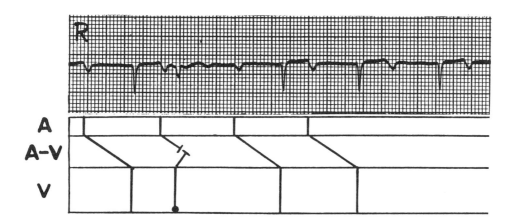

DIAGNOSIS: Sinus rhythm with first degree A-V block (P-R = 0.54 s)—sinus P waves are of course normally inverted in lead aVR. One premature beat, presumably ventricular.

SPECIAL POINTS: The extrasystole has a seemingly narrow QRS and could be junctional with aberrant conduction; but ventricular extrasystoles are much more common and quite often are small and narrow-looking in a single lead. The beat is followed by a slightly-less-than-fully compensatory cycle: not because the premature beat is supraventricular, but because, following the early beat, the longer R-P is naturally complemented by a slightly shorter P-R (0.50 s).

TREATMENT: Although first degree A-V block almost never requires therapy, when the P-R interval is this long—so that the P wave is superimposed on the preceding T wave—there is probably no atrial kick as atrial contraction has probably occurred before the A-V valves have opened. If, for this hemodynamic reason, it is desirable to shorten the P-R interval to restore the atrial transport function, atropine or isoproterenol may be indicated.

22. From a 60-year old white woman with a history of anterior infarction three years ago; she has severe angina of effort and is receiving propranolol and diltiazem.

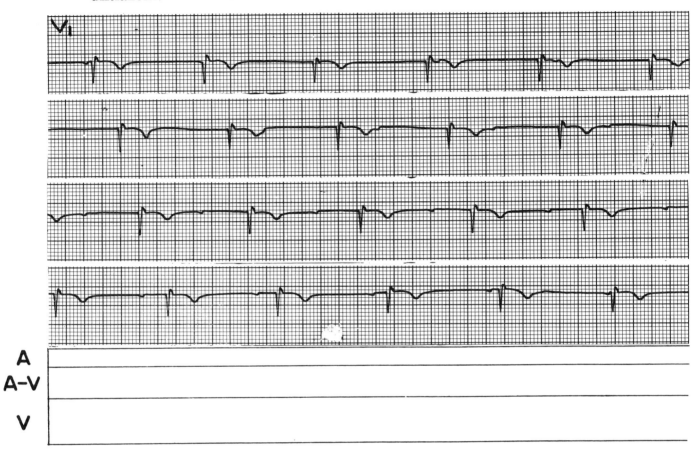

A

A-V

V

#22 DIAGNOSIS: Complete A-V dissociation due to A-V block. The atrial rate is 47/min and the ventricular rate 49-50/min.

SPECIAL POINTS: The P wave marches steadily across the R-R interval, but the atrial impulse never captures the ventricles. All phases of the cardiac cycle are probed by the atrial impulse, no conduction occurs and therefore the block is probably complete. However, most authorities require a ventricular rate under 45 before making the diagnosis of complete A-V block—some even require a rate under 40/min. Another claim that is sometimes—erroneously—made is that in complete A-V block the atrial rate is necessarily faster than the ventricular; and, of course, in most cases this is true. But, in fact, the atrial rate is irrelevant provided the other three criteria are satisfied: 1) no conduction in the presence of 2) a slow enough ventricular rate (40-45), and 3) the atrial impulse probing all phases of the cardiac cycle. In this case, because of the ventricular rate, we must be content to call it complete A-V dissociation due to A-V block, rather than "complete" A-V block.

TREATMENT: This patient needs help: She has angina and bradycardia, and has been deprived of her atrial kick by medications. If a normal rate and A-V conduction could be restored, it might work wonders with her angina. An effort should be made to reduce or eliminate her bradycardia-inducing and block-provoking drugs. If necessary, her rate may have to be increased and her atrial transport function restored by installing a dual-chambered pacemaker.

23. From a 78-year old white man who suffers from both typical angina of effort and shortness of breath; he is on no medications.

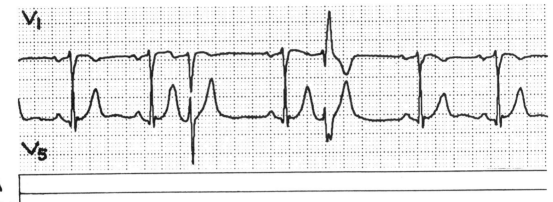

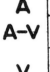

#23 DIAGNOSIS: Sinus rhythm with two aberrantly conducted atrial extrasystoles, the first with left anterior hemiblock aberration, the second with bifascicular (RBBB and left anterior hemiblock) aberration.

SPECIAL POINT: Note that anterior hemiblock causes little if any change in lead V1, but produces loss of q, shrinkage of R, and marked deepening of the S wave in V6.

TREATMENT: For a general approach to the treatment of atrial extrasystoles, see page 107.

24. From a 46-year old white diabetic woman admitted to CCU with retrosternal
    pain but without enzyme elevation. This rhythm strip was recorded shortly
    after admission. (The three strips are continuous).

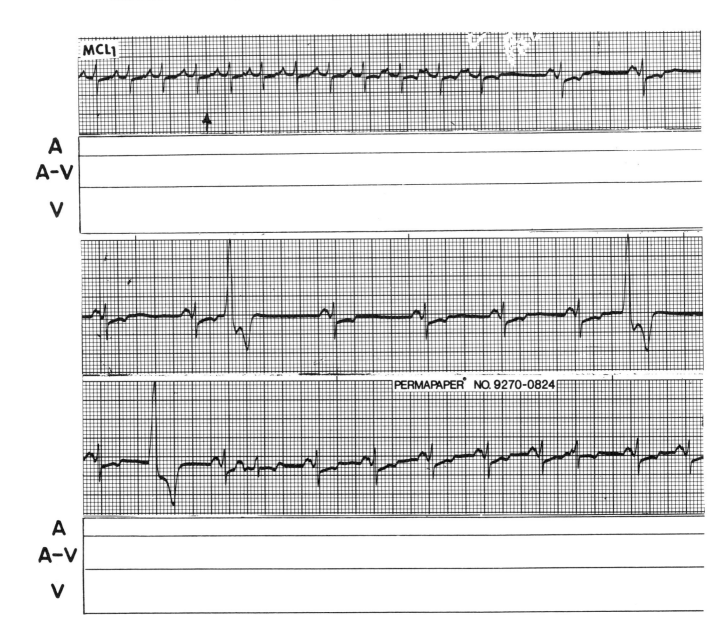

#24 **DIAGNOSIS:** Atrial tachycardia (rate 160/min) converted to sinus rhythm which is interrupted by ventricular and atrial premature beats.

SPECIAL POINTS: Note that the three VPBs all have different coupling intervals. This always raises the question of parasystole—so put your calipers to work and measure the interectopic intervals! In this case it does not measure out—the longer interectopic interval is not a multiple of the shorter.

TREATMENT: In this patient, carotid sinus massage was initiated at the arrow two minutes after 1 mg of propranolol had been given intravenously. For a general approach to the treatment of supraventricular tachycardia, see page 109.

25. From a 16-year old girl with hyperthyroidism, whose family physician prescribed digoxin because of a heart rate of 110/min. She complains of pulsations in her neck and "skipped beats."

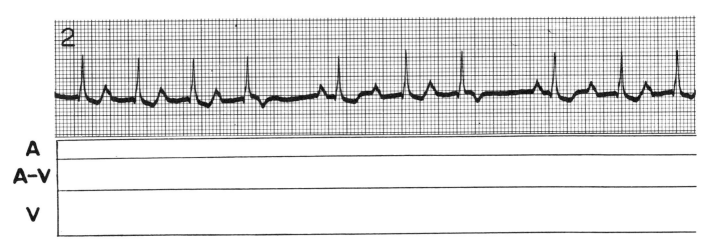

A

A-V

V

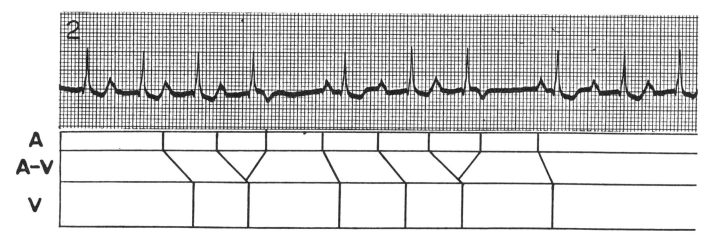

DIAGNOSIS: Sinus tachycardia with developing Wenckebach periods interrupted and aborted by reversed reciprocal beating (atrial "echoes"—see laddergram). The ST-T pattern, looking like an inverted check mark, is typical of digitalis effect.

SPECIAL POINT: This is a beautiful example of the importance of delayed conduction in initiating reentry. The inverted P waves might easily be mistaken for nonconducted atrial premature beats; but they are clearly dependent upon a critical degree of A-V delay (P-R prolongation), which identifies them as offspring of reentry.

TREATMENT: Discontinue digoxin and initiate appropriate antithyroid therapy.

26. From the same patient as #20, now aware of his slow heart beat.

52

#26 **DIAGNOSIS:** Complete A-V block with junctional escape rhythm at rate 43/min and rate-dependent LBBB; one ventricular extrasystole in each lead.

SPECIAL POINTS: It would be impossible to determine whether the independent ventricular rhythm was junctional with BBB or idioventricular if it were not for the post-extrasystolic escape beats. These returning beats, with their narrower QRSs ending the longer cycles, clearly suggest that the ventricular rhythm is supraventricular with BBB rather than ectopic ventricular. Note that the post-extrasystolic beat in lead aVF could easily escape notice because it is perched on a P wave and is, itself, of the shape and small size that might be mistaken for a P wave.

TREATMENT: A permanent pacemaker is still clearly indicated!

27. From a 48-year old man, a known hypertensive for six years, who is receiving hydrochlorothiazide and propranolol; he has no symptoms except for occasional headaches, and his blood pressure is now 145/88.

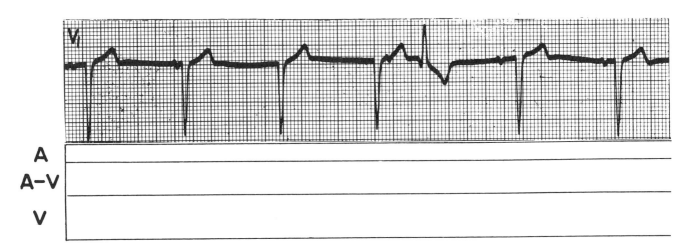

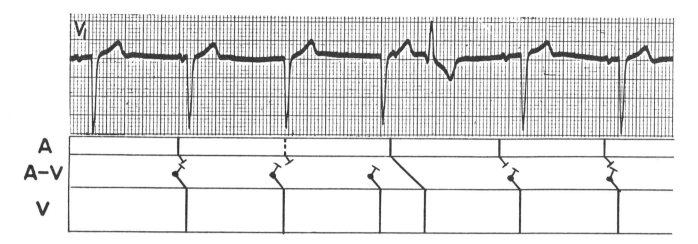

DIAGNOSIS: Sinus bradycardia (rate 52/min) with resulting junctional escape and A-V dissociation; one ventricular capture with prolonged P-R and RBBB aberration.

SPECIAL POINTS: Whenever A-V dissociation is diagnosed, one must determine the cause, because dissociation itself is but a symptom. The four causes of A-V dissociation are: 1) sinus bradycardia; 2) blockade of the sinus impulse (SA block or A-V block); 3) acceleration of a subsidiary pacemaker (accelerated junctional or ventricular rhythm, junctional or ventricular tachycardia); and 4) pause-producers (generally extrasystoles).

In this case, the primary cause is sinus bradycardia, although the junctional escape rate borders on "accelerated" (56/min). The long P-R interval in the conducted beat indicates that delayed A-V conduction is also present—but this plays no causative role in the A-V dissociation here.

TREATMENT: As always, in all forms of A-V dissociation, treatment—if needed—is directed at the underlying cause of the dissociation. Here it is due to the sinus bradycardia, no doubt in turn caused by the propranolol. In this case, therapy—as it so often does—requires a balancing act: The value of the drug in control of his hypertension versus the disadvantages, if any, of a rate of only 58 and the presence of A-V dissociation. Since the patient appears not to be compromised by his arrhythmia and his blood pressure is well controlled, leaving well enough alone is probably prudent.

28. From a 17-year old athletic boy with no complaints. At the time of a school physical, cannon waves were noted in the neck and this ECG was taken. (The strips are continuous).

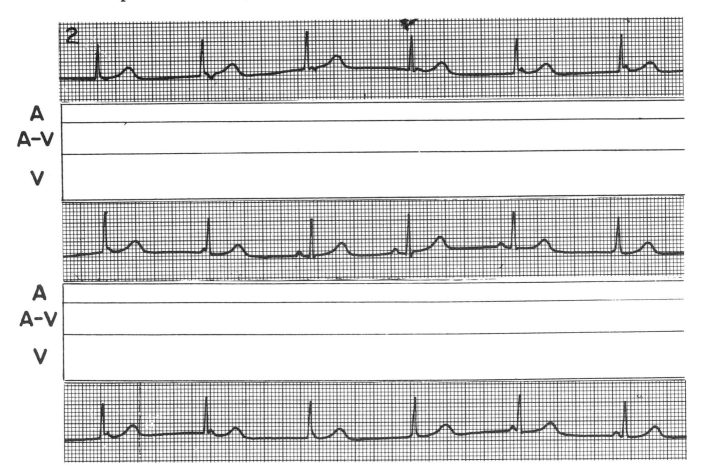

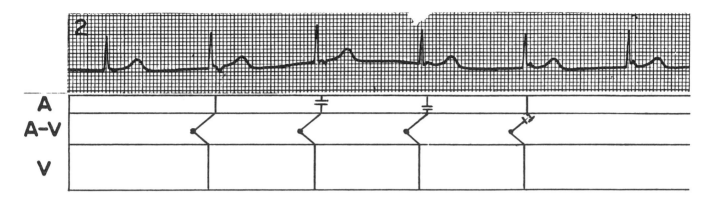

DIAGNOSIS: Junctional rhythm at rate 52 with sometimes retrograde conduction, sometimes A-V dissociation. On one occasion there is atrial fusion (P waves after third and fourth QRS's in top strip—see laddergram) and there is one conducted sinus beat (fourth beat in second strip).

SPECIAL POINTS: The fact that A-V conduction is successful in the middle of the second strip is recognized, not by the normal-looking P-R interval, but by the fact that the <u>ventricular cycle</u> measurably and momentarily shortens.

Since the independent sinus and junctional rates are virtually identical, the dissociation may be called "isorhythmic." Obviously there is an underlying sinus bradycardia—otherwise the junction would not be able to hold sway at a rate of 52/min.

TREATMENT: Clearly no therapy is indicated.

29. From a 53-year old woman with rheumatic heart disease, aware that her heart was beating irregularly.

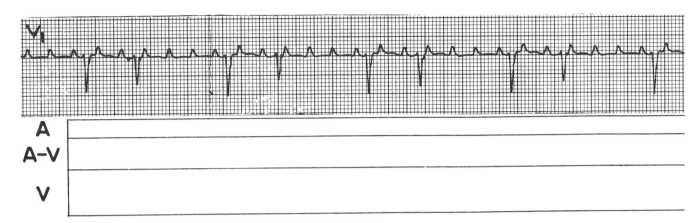

A

A–V

V

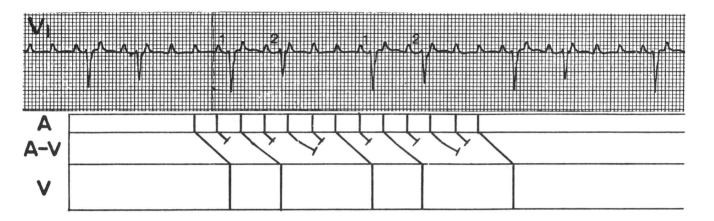

DIAGNOSIS: Atrial flutter with alternating 4:1 and 2:1 A-V conduction, because of 2:1 conduction at an upper level in the A-V junction with 3:2 Wenckebachs at a lower level (see laddergram).

SPECIAL POINT: When 4:1 and 2:1 conduction alternate in atrial flutter, it is invariably due to Wenckebach-type conduction at a lower level with a 2:1 "filter" at an upper level in the A-V junction. You can always spot it by looking at the A-V interval immediately in front of the paired ventricular complexes—the second (2) is always longer than the first (1). But note (see laddergram) that the atrial impulse that actually evokes the ventricular response is not the flutter wave immediately in front of the QRS, but the one before that—it is thought that the conducted F-R intervals in atrial flutter (as measured from the nadir of the flutter wave to the beginning of the QRS) are generally between 0.26 and 0.45 s.

TREATMENT: The flutter could of course be easily converted electrically, but since the situation is not urgent, a prudent approach would be to further slow the ventricular response to a constant 4:1 conduction with digitalis, propranolol or verapamil. With the better perfusion achieved with a normal ventricular rate, the arrhythmia may convert without further intervention. For a general approach to the treatment of atrial flutter, see page 110.

30. From a young man of 18 years with rheumatic aortic stenosis and regurgitation, conscious of vigorous pulsation in his neck.

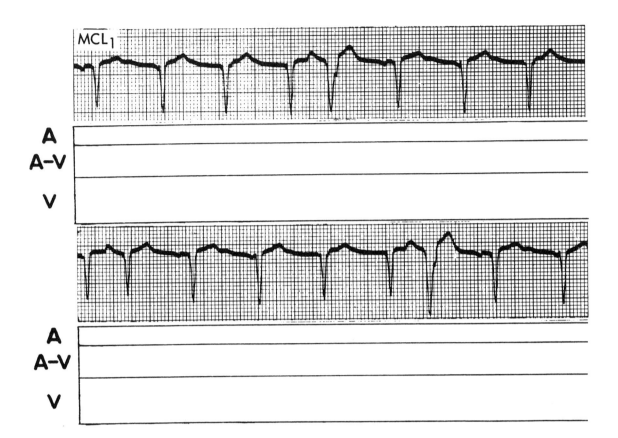

#30 **DIAGNOSIS:** Accelerated idiojunctional rhythm (rate 84/min) dissociated from the sinus rhythm (rate 72/min), with three ventricular captures, two of them with LBBB aberration.

SPECIAL POINTS: The aberrantly conducted captured beats might easily be mistaken for ventricular extrasystoles; but they show the typical morphology for LBBB, namely, a slick downstroke to an early nadir with slurring on the upstroke; and they are constantly related to an antecedent P wave deforming the ST segment. The second capture beat (second beat in bottom strip) is not aberrant because it ends a slightly longer cycle than the other aberrant ones.

TREATMENT: The arrhythmia itself demands no therapy, unless the loss of atrial transport function is hemodynamically embarrassing; but one should make sure that the accelerated subsidiary rhythm is not due to a recurrence of acute rheumatism.

31. From a 26-year old woman with a history of paroxysms of rapid heart beating since the age of ten years. (The three lead-tiers are simultaneous).

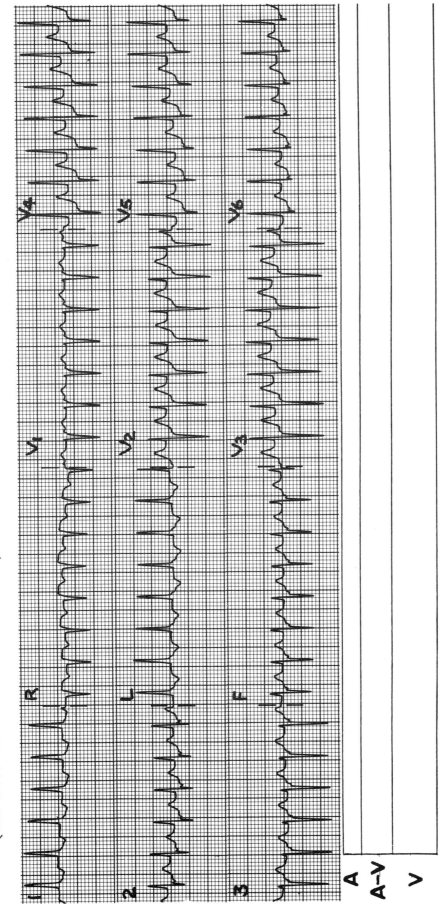

#31 DIAGNOSIS: Supraventricular tachycardia, almost certainly A-V nodal reentrant.

SPECIAL POINT: In the common form ("slow-fast") of A-V nodal reentrant tachycardia, the circulating wave uses the fast (beta) track for the retrograde journey to the atria and so the retrograde P wave occurs simultaneously—or almost simultaneously—with the QRS complex. The P wave is therefore either completely invisible within the QRS complex, or—as in this case—just peeping out at the end of the QRS, looking like an s wave in lead 2 and an r in V1.

TREATMENT: This tachycardia may terminate spontaneously, respond to rest or vagal maneuvers, or perhaps require intervention with an I-V dose of verapamil or a bolus of adenosine.

32. From a 56-year old man with rheumatic mitral regurgitation, receiving no medications.

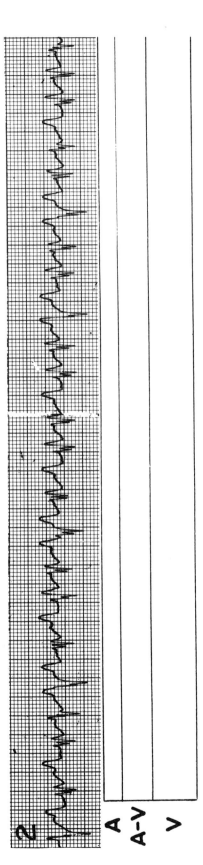

A

A–V

V

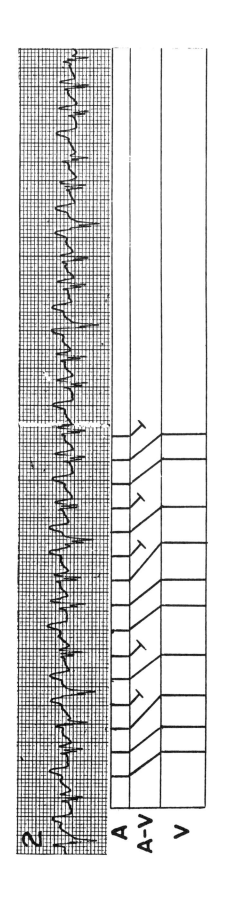

#32 **DIAGNOSIS:** Atrial tachycardia (rate 230/min) with 2:1 A-V conduction and 4:3 and 3:2 Wenckebach periods (see laddergram).

SPECIAL POINT: The apparent beat-to-beat change in the size and shape of the QRS's is entirely due to their constantly changing relationship to the sizeable P waves of opposite polarity.

TREATMENT: Therapy must be directed at slowing the ventricular rate either by converting the tachycardia, or by reducing the number of conducted beats by increasing A-V block. In the presence of congestive heart failure the treatment of choice is I-V digoxin. Rapid control of the ventricular rate could be obtained with verapamil or propranolol and this would probably outweigh their negative inotropic effects.

For a general approach to the treatment of supraventricular tachycardias, see page 109.

33. From a 36-year old multipara who developed heart failure during her third pregnancy one year ago. She was digitalized, her failure improved and she was maintained on 0.25 mg. of digoxin daily. Diuretics were added, with further improvement at first, but then her condition slowly deteriorated and this rhythm strip was obtained at an out-patient visit.

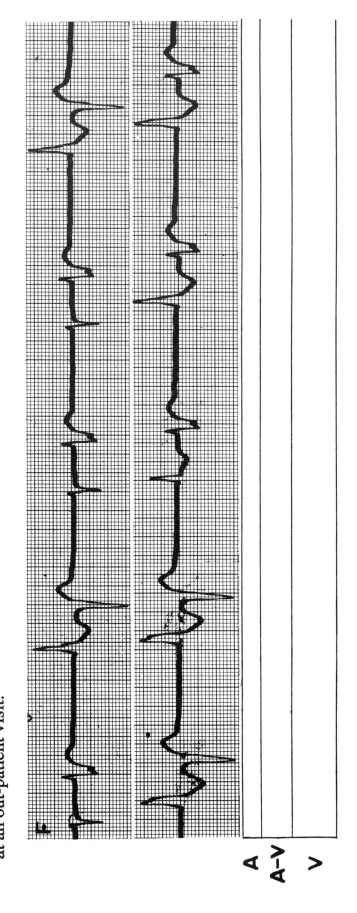

A

A–V

V

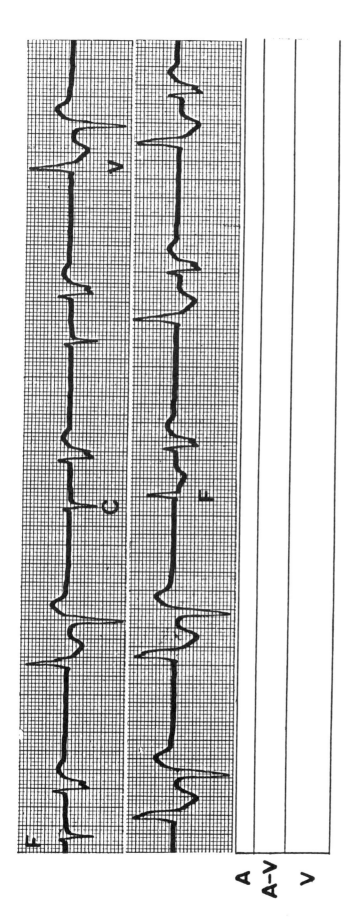

#33 DIAGNOSIS: "Straight-line" atrial fibrillation with significant A-V block. The long cycles sometimes end with conduction to the ventricles ('C'—narrow, negative QRS's ending somewhat shorter cycles); but more often with ventricular escape beats ('V'—wider, positive QRS's ending somewhat longer cycles); in bottom strip, the 5th beat ('F') is probably a fusion beat between a conducted impulse and a ventricular escape; ventricular bigeminy from two ectopic foci.

SPECIAL POINT: The combination of A-V block with multiform ventricular bigeminy is extremely suspicous of digitalis intoxication, which of course is the culprit here.

TREATMENT: Clearly the most important measure is to discontinue dogoxin.

34. From a child of 6 years who developed rheumatic fever two weeks after a severe sore throat was treated with penicillin. These rhythm strips were recorded on his third hospital day.

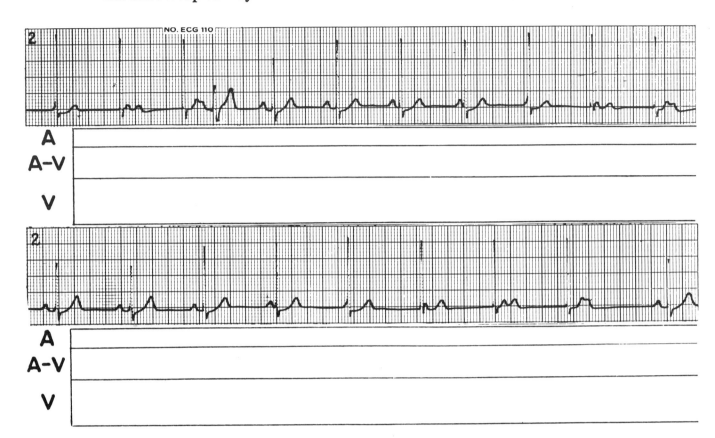

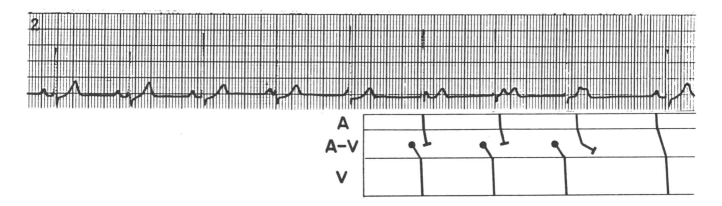

34

DIAGNOSIS: Accelerated junctional rhythm, dissociated from a slightly slower sinus rhythm, with one ventricular capture showing aberration (fourth beat in top strip); on one occasion towards the end of the bottom strip, concealed conduction of a sinus impulse discharges the junctional pacemaker and permits the sinus to regain control (see laddergram); minor aberration of junctional beats.

SPECIAL POINT: Note the difference in the QRS of conducted sinus beats and of junctional beats: The junctional beats have distinctly taller R waves. Slight differences in the QRS-T of junctional beats are explained by assuming that they often originate from a focus situated somewhat eccentrically in the A-V junction; and therefore, compared to the sinus impulses, they are distributed to the ventricles somewhat differently.

TREATMENT: The arrhythmia itself requires no therapy—it will abate with resolution of the rheumatic fever.

35. From a 69-year old black man with severe retrosternal pain admitted to the CCU five hours before this tracing was obtained. The pain was controlled with Innovar and at the time of this tachycardia he was pain-free with blood pressure 122/74. A 75 mg. bolus of lidocaine has failed to convert the tachycardia.

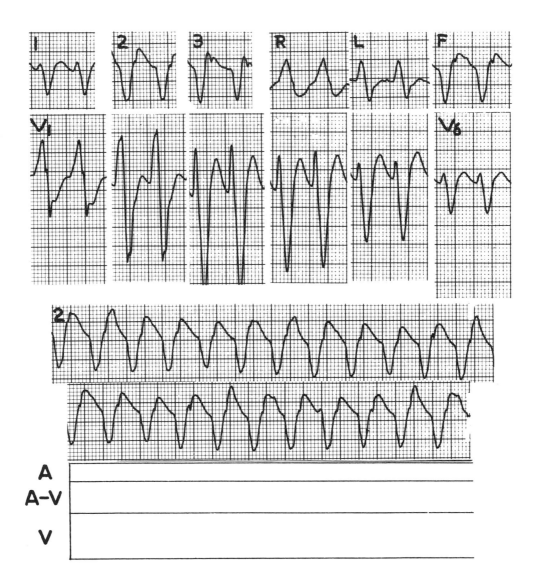

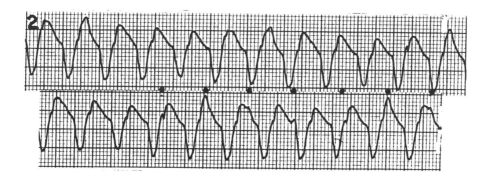

35

DIAGNOSIS: Left ventricular tachycardia.

SPECIAL POINTS: The morphological features that are typical for ventricular ectopy rather than aberration are: 1) a frontal plane axis in no-man's land (right upper quadrant); 2) RS complex in V1 and V2 with interval to nadir of S more than 0.10 s; 3) rS complex in V6. In addition, there is the compelling clue of dissociated atrial activity—independent P waves in the bottom strip are indicated by superposed dots.

TREATMENT: In the presence of presumed myocardial infarction, ventricular tachycardia that has not responded to a tentative bolus of lidocaine should be promptly terminated by DC cardioversion—ventricular tachycardia of recent origin usually responds to a small dose of 10-20 joules.

36. From a 76-year old man with ischemic heart disease and severe mitral regurgitation from papillary muscle dysfunction. (The strips are not continuous).

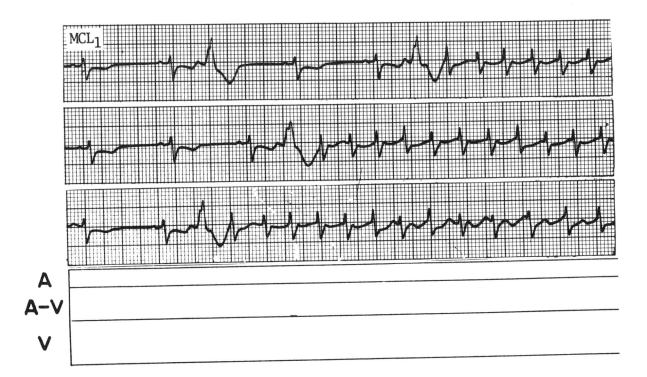

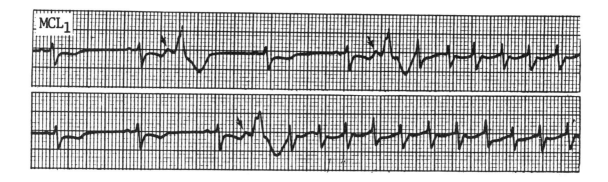

36

DIAGNOSIS: Sinus rhythm with atrial prematrue beats conducted with RBBB aberration and precipitating an irregular atrial tachyarrhythmia.

SPECIAL POINTS: Whenever the second-in-a-row of rapid beats is anomalous, there are always two possibilities: That the QRS is aberrant (since it is the only beat ending a short cycle preceded by a significantly longer cycle), or a VPB with retrograde conduction initiating a reentrant tachycardia. In this case, the QRS morphology of the anomalous beat is not diagnostic, but close inspection reveals that each anomalous complex is preceded by a premature P wave (arrows); this clinches the diagnosis of APBs with RBBB aberration.

TREATMENT: For a general approach to the treatment of supraventricular tachyarrhythmias, see page 109.

37. From a 24-year old man with mitral regurgitation receiving no medication. He has had repeated bouts of rapid heart beating for the past several years. (The strips are not continuous).

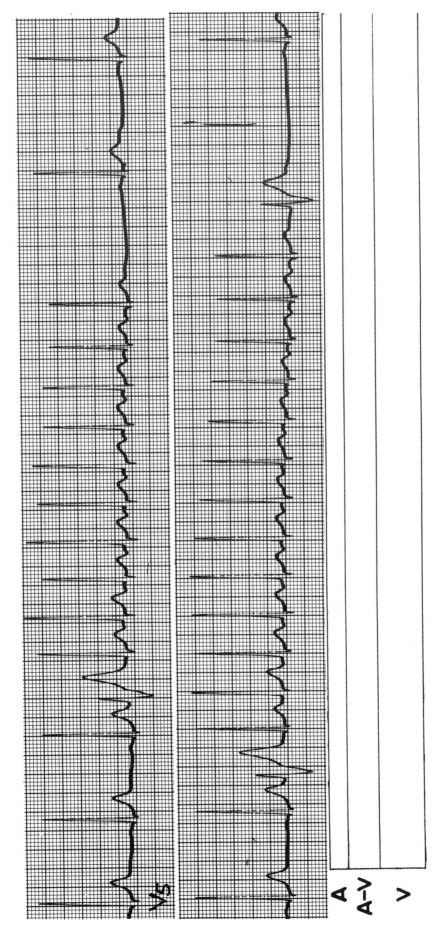

V5

A

A–V

V

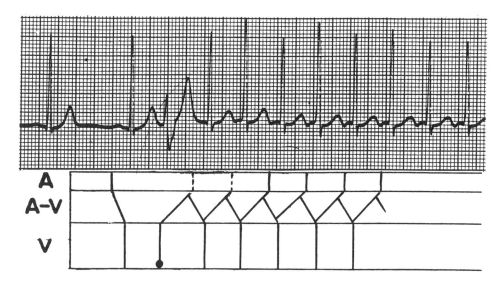

37

DIAGNOSIS: Sinus rhythm interrupted by ventricular extrasystoles that initiate runs of reentrant A-V tachycardia (see laddergram); overdrive suppression of sinus node.

SPECIAL POINTS: The reentrant tachycardia is probably an othodromic, circus-movement tachycardia, using a slowly conducting accessory pathway for the retrograde journey—because the R-P′ is greater than the P′-R interval; it could, of course, be the relatively rare "fast-slow" A-V nodal reentrant tachycardia.

When the second-in-a-row of rapid beats is wide and bizarre, one must always think of aberration; and here the shape of the anomalous beats (absent q, shrunken R and deep, wide S wave) might well be bifascicular (RBBB + left anterior hemiblock) aberration; but here the evidence against aberration is in the third anomalous beat—the penultimate complex in the bottom strip—which ends a cycle distinctly longer than the cycle during the tachycardia and thus has no reason to be aberrant. The probability is, therefore, that the anomalous beats are ectopic ventricular.

The slowed sinus response at the end of each strip after the paroxysm is the result of repeated rapid depolarization of the sinus node by the retrograde atrial impluses ("overdrive suppression").

TREATMENT: For a general approach to the treatment of supraventricular tachycardias, see page 109.

38. This 34-year old Indian woman has an accentuated first heart sound and a rumbling middiastolic murmur; she has mild dyspnea on effort and is receiving digoxin 0.25 mg. daily. (The strips are continuous).

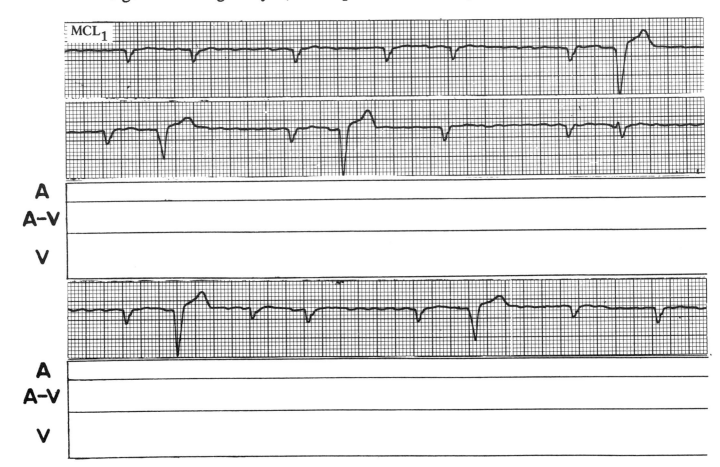

#38 **DIAGNOSIS:** Atrial fibrillation with controlled ventricular response and probably incomplete LBBB; frequent ventricular extrasystoles (from at least two foci) obeying the "rule of bigeminy."

SPECIAL POINTS: This illustrates well the dependence of some extrasystoles on the preceding cycle length. In this tracing, only cycles of 1.28 s or longer are followed by an ectopic beat.

When digitalis causes ventricular premature beats, the QRS is said to be never uniform; here the configuration of the last beat in the second strip is obviously quite different from all the other extrasystoles.

TREATMENT: Very likely no treatment is necessary; but, since it is possible that the long precipitating cycles and the ventricular extrasystoles are both caused by digitalis, it would be prudent to observe the effect of reducing or temporarily discontinuing the drug.

For a general approach to the treatment of atrial fibrillation, see page 111.

39. From a 55-year old white man who sustained a myocardial infarction the day before this rhythm strip was recorded. At the time of this tracing, his blood pressure was 110/68 and he was asymptomatic. (The strips are continuous).

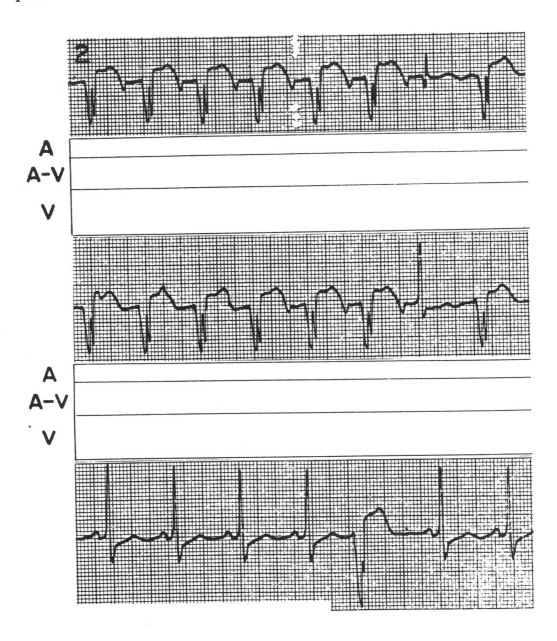

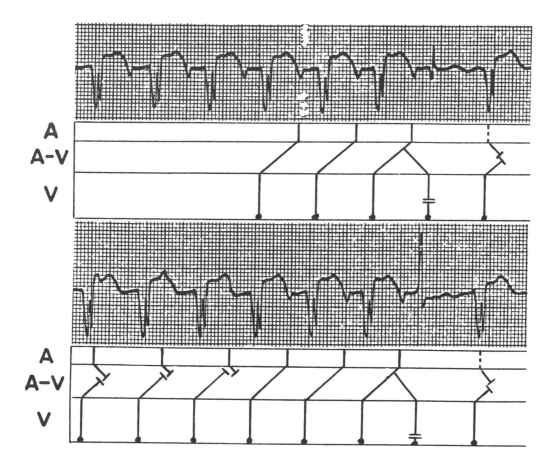

DIAGNOSIS: Ventricular tachycardia (rate 100/min) with retrograde conduction to atria and reciprocal beating producing fusion beats. Following the first fusion beat, four ventricular beats are dissociated from sinus P waves before retrograde conduction resumes. One VPB interrupts sinus rhythm in the bottom strip.

SPECIAL POINTS: The fusion beats are interesting: first of all, we know they are not pure reciprocal beats because their QRS's differ from those of the conducted sinus beats in the bottom strip; and then both of them occur at exactly the moment that the next ectopic beat was due. They therefore represent fusion between the next ectopic beat of the tachycardia and the descending reciprocal impulse (see laddergram).

TREATMENT: At the rate of 100/min, this rhythm is teetering between accelerated idioventricular rhythm and ventricular tachycardia, and at this rate is not unduly dangerous. The patient tolerates it well, and it appears to be self-terminating; he should be vigilantly observed, but it is unlikely that agressive therapy will be required.

40. From a 64-year old white man with a ten-year history of angina and with dyspnea on effort for the past year; he is receiving diltiazem and a diuretic and is aware of intermittent palpitation. (The strips are continuous).

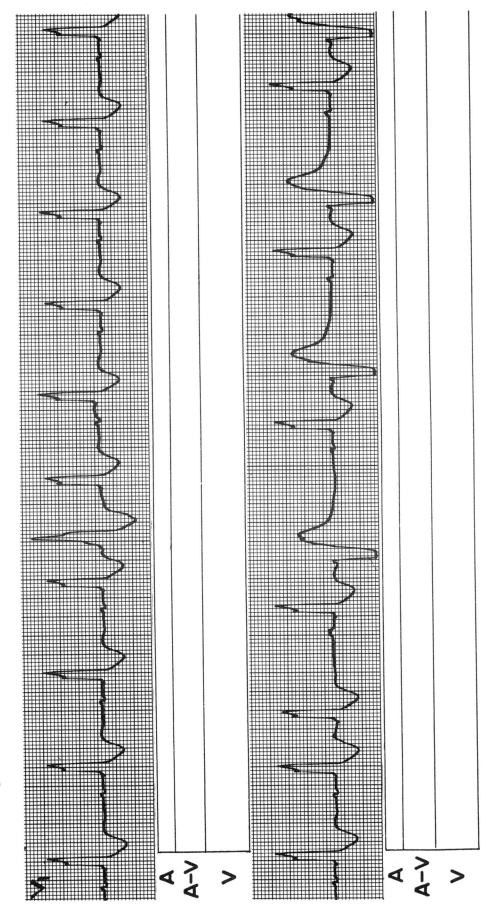

#40 **DIAGNOSIS:** Sinus rhythm with mild first degree A-V block (P-R = 0.22 s) and RBBB; interrupted by one left ventricular extrasystole, an atrial extrasystole, and four right ventricular extrasystoles in bigeminal rhythm.

SPECIAL POINTS: The left ventricular extrasystole has the typical early peak (taller left "rabbit-ear" equivalent) in constrast with the delayed peak in the RBBB beats.

The right ventricular bigeminy is initiated by the lengthened ventricular cycle produced by the atrial extraystole (overdrive suppression); it affords another good example of the "rule of bigeminy" in action (compare #s 20 and 38).

TREATMENT: It would clearly be desirable to eliminate the ectopic beats; but antiarrhythmic agents should be used with special caution in patients with BBB. Small doses of digoxin are quite safe in the presence of BBB, are quite effective against APBs (one of which is what precipitated the right ventricular bigeminy), and are often efficacious in the treatment of VPBs. Digoxin is therefore a reasonable, and perhaps the best, option.

41. From a 76-year old, overweight (216 lbs.) man with a 15-year history of hypertension, and progressive shortness of breath for the past three years. He was recently digitalized and is receiving 0.25 mg. digoxin b.i.d.

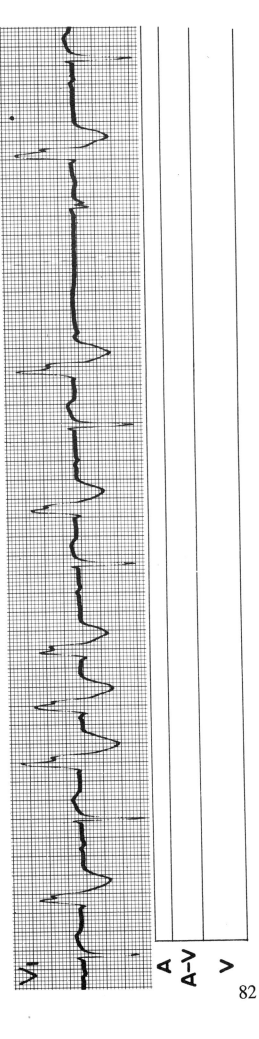

V₁

A
A–V
V

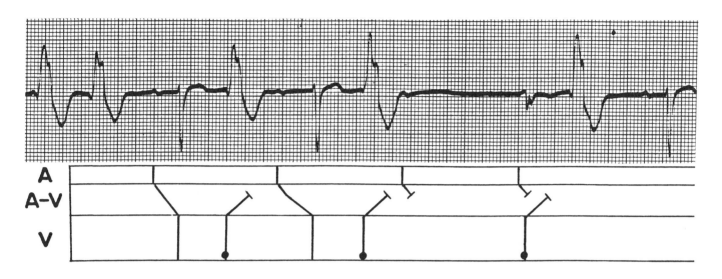

DIAGNOSIS: Sinus bradycardia (rate 45/min) interrupted by single left ventricular extrasystoles; and by one group of three such beats representing the shortest definable run of ventricular tachycardia; concealed retrograde conduction from the ectopic impulses produces P-R interval lengthening in the post-ectopic beats; one ventricular escape beat.

SPECIAL POINTS: Note the taller left "rabbit-ear" in the premature beats typical of left ventricular ectopy in V1.

When ventricular bigeminy is associated with concealed retrograde conduction—as in the two couplets following the trio of ectopic beats—a Wenckebach-like effect is produced by the progressively increasing effect of the successive retrograde conductions (see laddergram).

TREATMENT: These ventricular premature beats, being almost certainly secondary to digitalis overdosage, should be treated by reducing the dose or temporarily discontinuing the digoxin. Obviously, potassium levels should be checked and an intensive weight-reduction program instituted.

42. From a 75-year old diabetic and hypertensive man seen in the Emergency Room with cholecystitis. He has known coronary and peripheral vascular disease, and is taking atenolol and verapamil. (Tracing courtesy of David Spodick, M.D.)

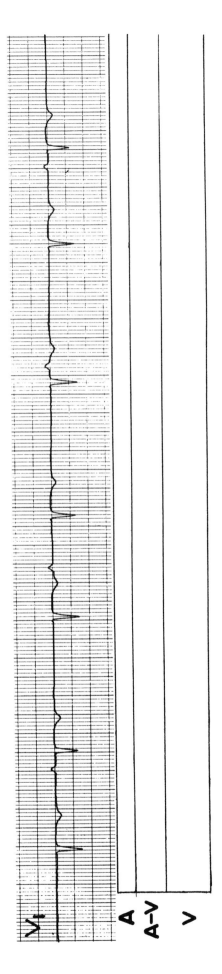

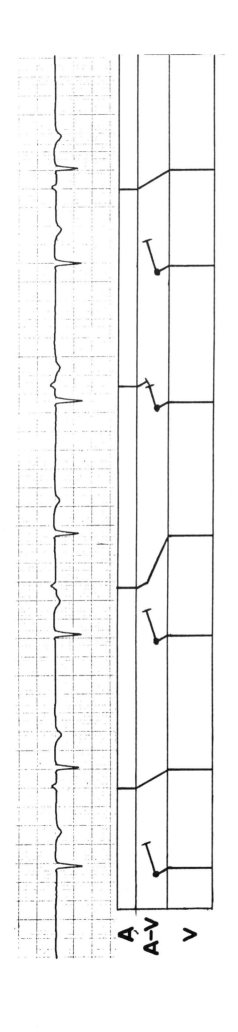

#42 **DIAGNOSIS:** Marked sinus bradycardia (rate = 43/min), permitting junctional escape at 28/min; the resulting A-V dissociation is interrupted by three ventricular captures manifesting R-P/P-R reciprocity.

SPECIAL POINT: The demonstrably reciprocal R-P/P-R relationship is evidence of a type I A-V nodal conduction defect.

TREATMENT: The primary diagnosis is a sick sinus (manifested by marked bradycardia) and that is what requires attention. If the cause is acute, atropine is appropriate therapy; if chronic, a permanent pacemaker. Most sick sinuses are best treated with an atrial pacemaker (AAI), but if there is evidence of impaired A-V conduction (as there is here), it would be prudent to employ a dual-chamber model.

43. From a 64-year old white woman with a history of ischemic heart disease, including angina at rest as well as on exertion. She is receiving nitroglycerin, diltiazem and isordil.

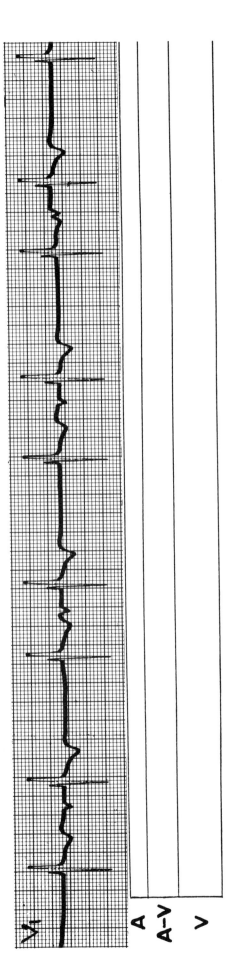

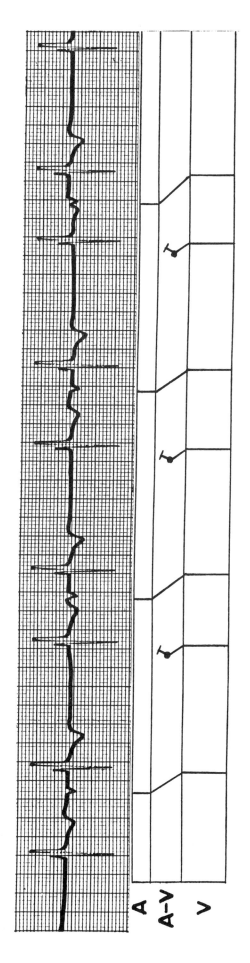

A

A-V

V

#43 **DIAGNOSIS:** Marked sinus bradycardia (rate 29/min) with junctional escape producing a form of "escape-capture" bigeminy, each pair consisting of a junctional escape followed by a conducted sinus beat with prolonged P-R interval (first degree A-V block). All beats show incomplete RBBB.

SPECIAL POINTS: In the differential diagnosis, reciprocal beating must be considered; but the great variability in the R-P interval makes it extremely unlikely that the P waves are retrogradely dependent on the preceding escape beat. Note that the R-P/P-R intervals manifest the typical reciprocity of type I A-V block.

TREATMENT: The primary diagnosis is clearly a sick sinus, and this is what must be addressed.

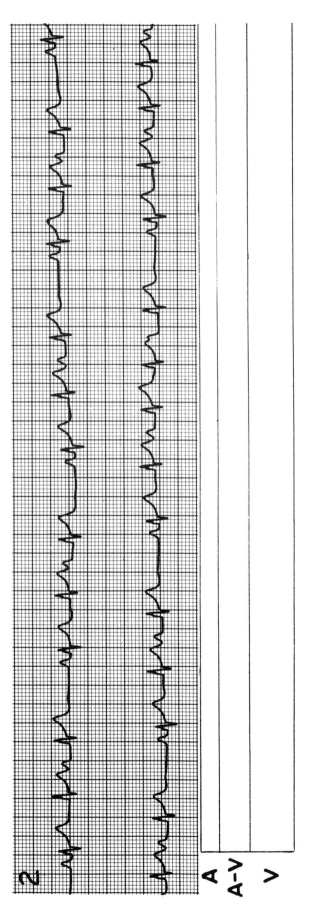

44. From an asymptomatic 15-year old boy. (The strips are not continuous).

88

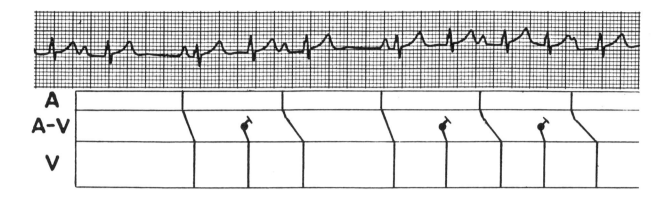

DIAGNOSIS: Sinus bradycardia (rate 56/min) with frequent interpolated junctional premature beats producing groups of three and five beats; following each interpolated extrasystole, the P-R interval of the ensuing sinus beat is prolonged (to about 0.24 s) because of nodal refractoriness in the extrasystole's aftermath (see laddergram).

TREATMENT: In an otherwise healthy asymptomatic youth, the arrhythmia is probably best left untreated. If treatment becomes necessary, the general approach to treating VPB's—outlined on page 106—should be followed.

45. From a 63-year old man with chest pain radiating down his right arm; this tracing was taken shortly after admission to the CCU.

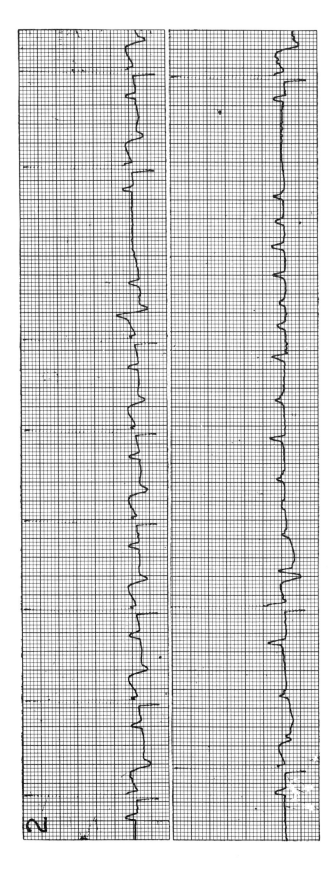

#45 **DIAGNOSIS:** Sinus rhythm with first degree A-V block (P-R = 0.25 s), interrupted by a pair of non-conducted atrial extrasystoles, and then by a six-second run of irregular, multifocal, atrial tachycardia; during the ectopic atrial activity, repetitive concealed conduction into the junction aggravates the mildly impaired A-V conduction and temporarily prevents all impulses from reaching the ventricles.

SPECIAL POINT: From the bottom strip, one might get the impression that the A-V block is severe (no A-V conduction for a five-second period); but from the top strip it is obvious that, at a normal atrial rate, A-V conduction is reasonably good (mild first degree A-V block). For the patient's sake, it is important to realize that in the presence of an atrial tachyarrhythmia (tachycardia, flutter or fibrillation) the block, because of the superimposed concealed conduction, may not be nearly as serious as it looks—get rid of the atrial tachycardia and the level of conduction may be quite acceptable.

TREATMENT: The first step in therapy is to understand the mechanisms involved and not to overreact to the seeming seriousness of the A-V block. In the absence of ectopic atrial activity, A-V conduction is only mildly disturbed and if one could eliminate the atrial ectopy—and with it the concealed conduction—A-V conduction would presumably be satisfactory. Digitalis, verapamil or propranolol might eliminate the ectopy, but also might aggravate the A-V block and therefore should probably be avoided; quinidine, on the other hand, is not only effective in eliminating atrial ectopy, but also (because of its antivagal effect) favors A-V conduction, and is therefore probably the drug of choice. If despite its use, the ectopy and the prolonged periods of ventricular asystole persist, a temporary pacemaker will be needed.

46. From a 56-year old woman with a permanent artificial pacemaker implanted a year ago for uncertain indications. She has been taking digoxin 0.25 mg. daily for the past two years. (The strips are continuous).

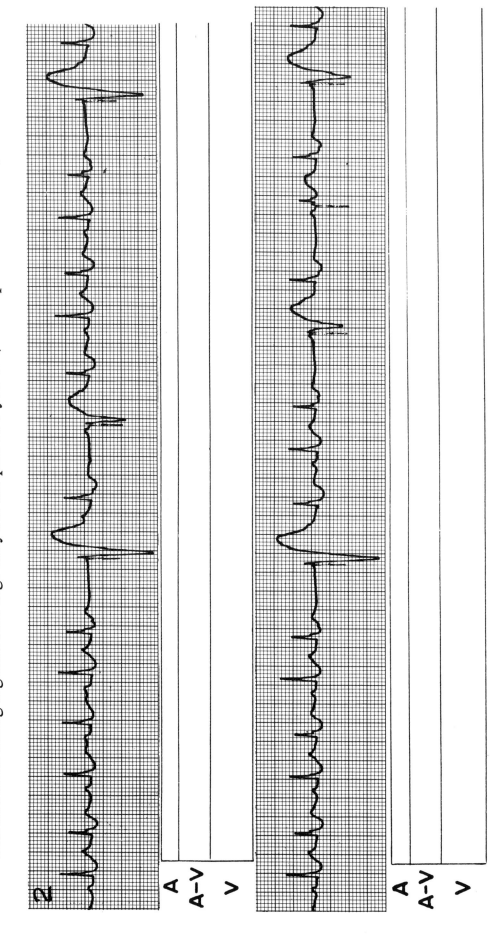

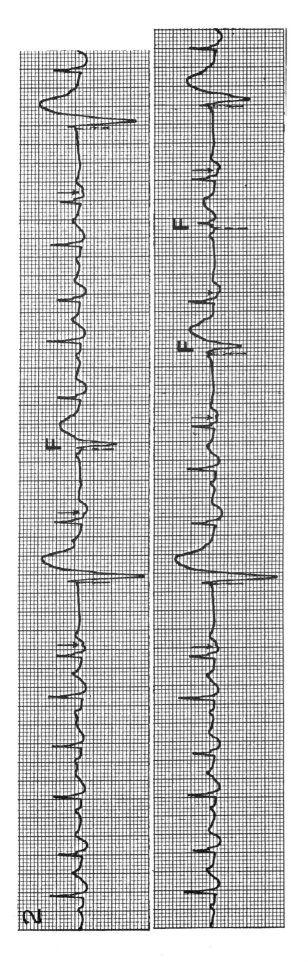

#46 **DIAGNOSIS:** Sinus rhythm with (mostly) atrial bigeminy; the demand pacemaker escapes only after a pair of atrial extrasystoles, the second of which (arrows) is non-conducted. Some paced impulses produce ventricular fusion (F).

TREATMENT: Atrial extrasystoles are sometimes an early sign of congestive heart failure; in a patient complaining of shortness of breath, digitalis is likely to be the tailor-made treatment—for a simultaneous antiarrhythmic and inotropic effect.

For a general approach to the treatment of atrial extrasystoles, see page 107.

93

47. From a 48-year old white woman in the CCU with acute anteroseptal infarction; at present she is not in pain, but is moderately short of breath and her blood pressure is 106/74. (The strips are not continuous).

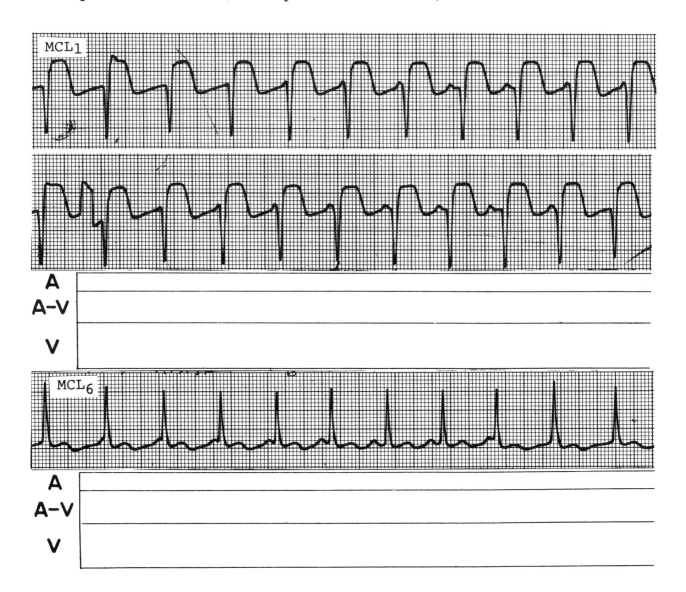

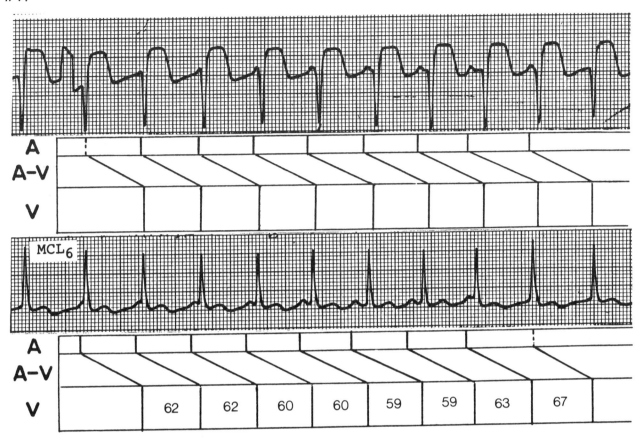

| | | | | 62 | 62 | 60 | 60 | 59 | 59 | 63 | 67 |

DIAGNOSIS: Sinus rhythm (rate 94/min) with first degree A-V block (P-R = 0.68-0.76 s)—see laddergram.

SPECIAL POINTS: In the differential diagnosis, one has to consider accelerated junctional rhythm dissociated from the sinus mechanism. But the evidence establishing conduction of all sinus impulses with prolonged P-Rs—the P-Rs sometimes longer than the R-Rs—is found in the subtle way that the ventricular rate parallels the atrial. For example, at the beginning of each strip (where the P wave is lost inside the QRS) the ventricular rate is measurably slower than when the atrial rate accelerates and P waves appear in front of the QRS—whereupon the ventricular cycles show parallel shortening. (Tracing #48 from the same patient further supports this interpretation).

TREATMENT: The A-V conduction defect is unimportant since it is obviously A-V nodal and since the ventricular rate is more than adequate. At this point clearly no effort should be made to treat the A-V block.

Sinus tachycardia is always of serious concern in the presence of acute myocardial infarction and it is important to look for contributory causes and elininate them if possible. Congestive failure, pulmonary emboli, complicating infections, should be looked for and dealt with. If one decides that temporary slowing of the sinus rate would be beneficial, intravenous esmolol is a possible option.

48. From the same patient as #47 several hours later. (The strips of MCL$_1$ are not continuous).

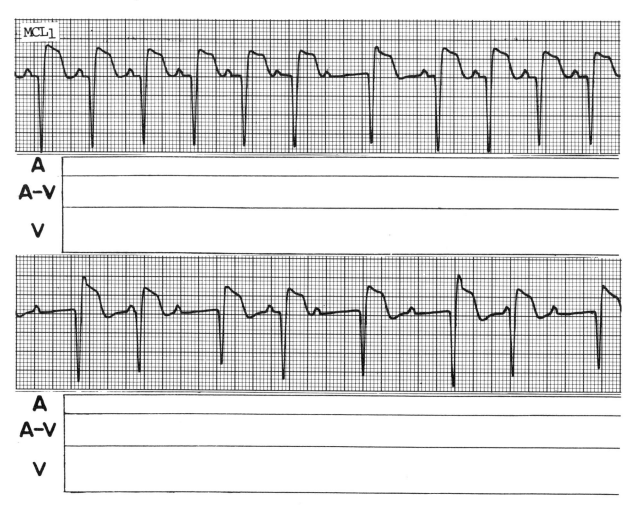

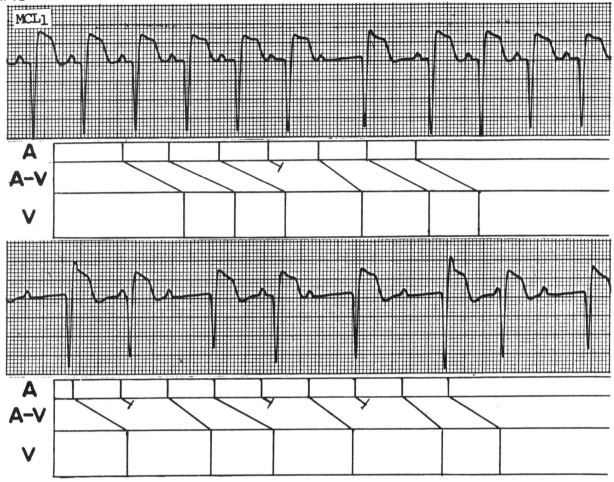

48

DIAGNOSIS: Sinus tachycardia (rate 110/min) with A-V Wenckebach periods and 2:1 conduction (see laddergram).

SPECIAL POINTS: These Wenckebach periods, in which many of the P-R intervals are longer than the R-R intervals, afford collateral evidence for the postulated conduction pattern in #47.

Some observers have difficulty in understanding that it is possible for an atrial impulse, whose P wave is in front of a QRS, to be conducted "over the top" of the QRS to the next one. But the difficulty stems from our habit of recording on two-dimensional paper events that are taking place at very different levels in the heart.

If the sinus node has orders to beat at 110/min, it will beat at that rate; and when the time comes for it to fire, it is of no concern whether or not the previous impulse has yet reached the ventricles—the sinus node has no reason to wait till the last impulse has reached its destination before it again discharges! And this irrelevance is immediately obvious if you look at the laddergram instead of at the tracing.

TREATMENT: Comments under #47 apply here.

49. From a 56-year old hypertensive man who had a cerebral hemorrhage and lost consciousness at home. This rhythm strip was recorded in the Emergency Room.

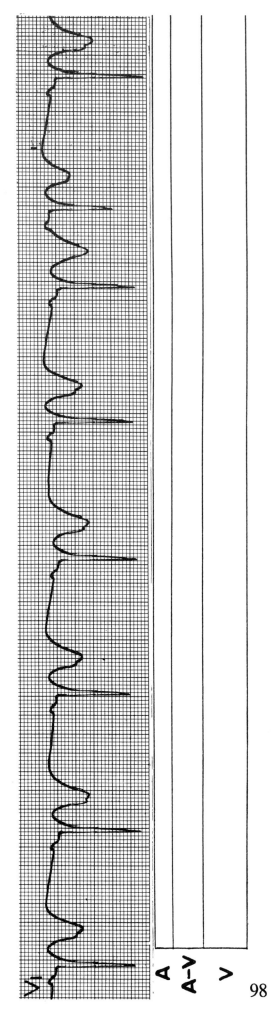

A

A–V

V

#49 **DIAGNOSIS:** Sinus rhythm with non-conducted atrial bigeminy.

SPECIAL POINTS: Non-conducted atrial bigeminy is the imitator of sinus bradycardia, and it would be easy to mistake the diagnosis here for sinus bradycardia interrupted by an atrial premature beat. The premature, non-conducted P' waves are obvious on close inspection of the nadirs of the plummeting T waves—compare with the smooth contour of the T wave preceding the sinus beat that ends the short cycle.

TREATMENT: Supportive therapy for the cerebrovascular accident is probably all that is therapeutically indicated.

For a general approach to the treatment of atrial extrasystoles, see page 107.

50. From a 73-year old black woman with aortic stenosis who had an anteroseptal infarction three years ago. She has recently complained of rapid, irregular heart beating; this rhythm strip was recorded in her physician's office.

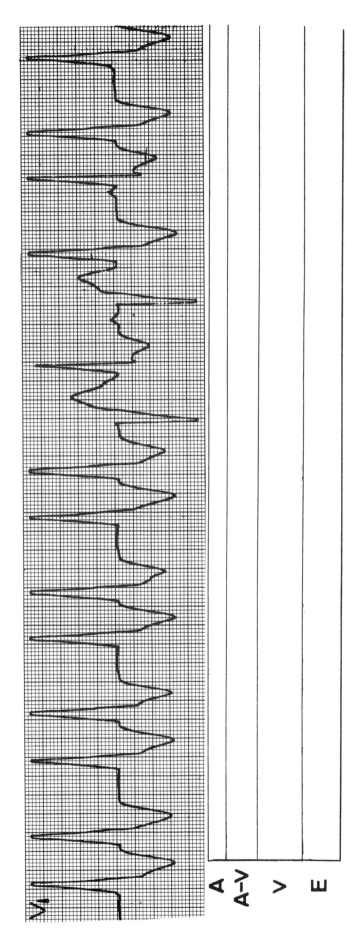

A
A–V
V
E

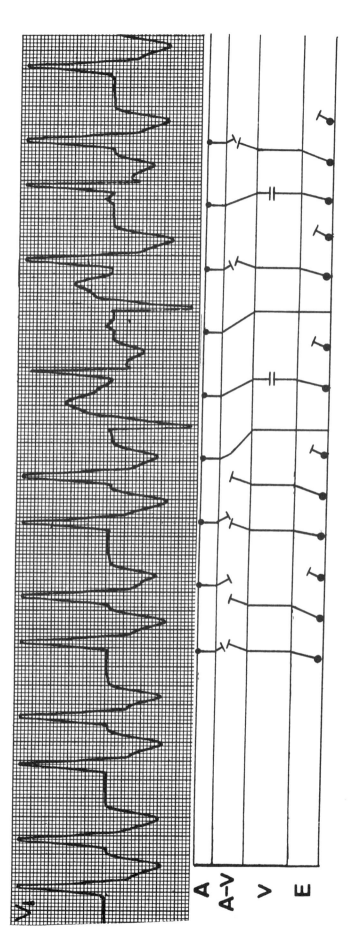

#50 DIAGNOSIS: Left ventricular tachycardia (discharge rate = 136/min, see laddergram) with 3:2 Wenckebach conduction out of the ectopic ventricular focus (E); two ventricular captures by the sinus with LBBB; two fusion beats.

SPECIAL POINTS: The grouping of the ectopic beats in pairs is a compelling clue to 3:2 Wenckebach-type conduction. Morphologically, note the tall single peak characteristic of some ectopic beats in V1, and in the conducted beats the slick downstroke with slurred upstroke so typical of LBBB. When fusion occurs between an ectopic impulse arising on the same side as a BBB, the fusion complex enjoys some measure of normalization—in this case the two fusion beats (10th and 13th beats), though far from normal, are slightly narrower than the "component" ectopic and conducted complexes.

TREATMENT: For a general approach to the treatment of ventricular tachycardia, see page 108.

51. From a 79-year old man with a history of bronchiectasis, old anterior infarction, hypertension and severe peripheral atherosclerosis with below-knee amputation of left leg; admitted to CCU after femoral-popliteal bypass surgery on other leg. (These selected strips are not continuous; tracing courtesy of Gail Ragsdale, R.N.).

MCL₁

#51 **DIAGNOSIS:** Sinus tachycardia (rate 114/min) with complete A-V dissociation due to A-V block; accelerated junctional and left ventricular rhythms at virtually identical rates (63-66)/min) producing numerous fusion beats (most of which simulate a RBBB pattern—rSR'). Isolated left ventricular extrasystoles in third and fourth strips; right ventricular extrasystoles, including one pair, but otherwise producing bigeminy in the top strip.

SPECIAL POINT: In the absence of all A-V conduction, it is not unusual to find a pair of independent, subsidiary pacemakers with virtually identical rates; and in these circumstances, an infinite variety of fusion QRS contours can result.

TREATMENT: In this patient's parlous state, there is probably little to be gained by attempting to suppress his VPBs; and certainly nothing is at present needed for his A-V block, since he has not one, but two active, natural pacemakers with satisfactory rates!

For a general approach to the treatment of VPBs, see page 106; and for A-V block, see page 113.

103

52. From an alert, apparently healthy, 80-year old man, who noted that his heart beat was "twinning"; this rhythm strip was recorded in the Emergency Room.

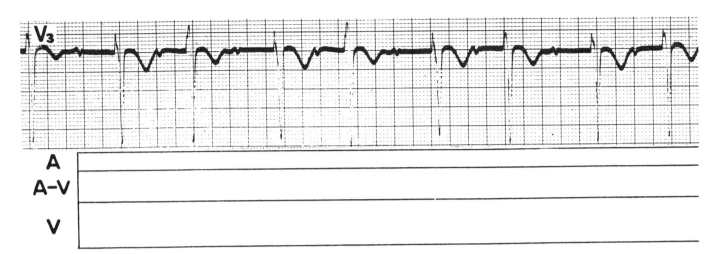

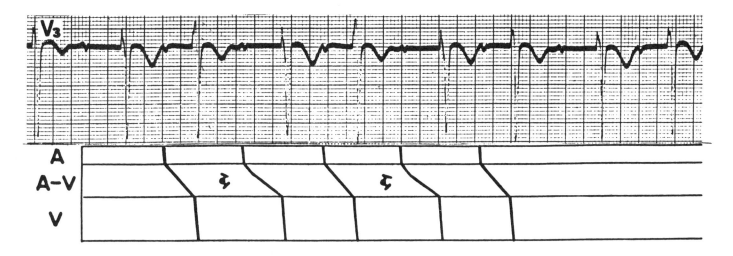

DIAGNOSIS: Sinus rhythm with first degree A-V block and bigeminal grouping produced by alternating P-R intervals (approximately 0.45 and 0.32 s)—probably caused by concealed junctional extrasystoles every third beat.

SPECIAL POINT: When A-V nodal conduction is impaired, there is usually a reciprocal relationship between the R-P and the P-R— the longer the R-P the shorter the P-R and vice versa (see #s 4, 9, 42, and 43). Here it is the opposite: The longer R-P is complemented by the longer P-R, and the shorter R-P by the shorter P-R. It used to be thought that "supernormal conduction" explained the improved A-V conduction after the shorter R-P, until Langendorf suggested the alternative and more likely explanation of concealed junctional extrasystoles (see laddergram).

TREATMENT: Extensive experience in treatment of junctional extrasystoles is lacking and one follows the general approach to the treatment of VPB's, see page 106.

GENERAL APPROACH TO TREATMENT OF VENTRICULAR EXTRASYSTOLES

In general, ventricular premature beats (VPB's) should go untreated. This is certainly true in the normal or near normal heart, no matter how frequent and numerous. Probably the only situations in which they should be treated are if they are causing intolerable palpitations that reassurance fails to soothe; in the presence of acute myocardial infarction; or in special circumstances where they pose a peculiar threat, as in hypokalemia or digitalis intoxication. Even with satisfactory suppression of VPBs in the sick heart, there is no convincing evidence that life is prolonged, and in some circumstances it may be shortened by the well-intentioned therapy.

The common sense approach to therapy may be summarized as follows:

1. Most VPBs should be left alone—treatment may be more dangerous than the extrasystoles. The only completely safe measure is the removal of recognized irritants, if any, such as caffeine, nicotine, etc.

2. If treatment is thought necessary, first try mild nonspecific sedatives or tranquillizers. If these fail and patient is very symptomatic, try propranolol, mexiletine, or moricizine.

3. For specific situations—if treatment is needed—certain drugs are appropriate, for example:

   a) if due to emotion or exertion: propranolol

   b) in acute myocardial infarction: lidocaine, procainamide

   c) if due to digitalis: withhold digitalis; additional therapy

      (potassium, propranolol or phenytoin) is unlikely to be needed

   d) in mitral valve prolapse: propranolol

4. Remember that digoxin in maintenance dosage is safe and often effective in eliminating VPBs (unless due to digitalis).

GENERAL APPROACH TO TREATMENT OF ATRIAL EXTRASYSTOLES (APBs)

APBs, often found in normal as well as diseased hearts, usually require no therapy. In the normal subject, reassurance is important and all that is necessary. If they become symptomatically troublesome, or trigger atrial tachyarrhythmias, one should attempt suppression: Avoid possible irritants, like caffeine, cigarettes, alcohol, etc.; try a sedative or tranquillizer; if necessary, move to stronger measures including digoxin, disopyramide or propranolol.

If there is any underlying disease, obviously its treatment is paramount. APBs are sometimes an early sign of congestive heart failure—in such cases, digoxin is the drug of choice.

GENERAL APPROACH TO TREATMENT OF VENTRICULAR TACHYCARDIA (VT)

Four out of five wide-QRS tachycardias are ectopic ventricular; because of this statistical fact, and because of the hazards of using verapamil in unrecognized VT, wide-QRS tachycardias should be treated as VT unless there is overwhelming evidence in favor of ventricular aberration.

Although VT is almost the monopoly of the diseased heart, very brief (3- or 4-beat) runs are occasionally encountered in normal or near-normal hearts in 24-hour recordings; if asymptomatic, the subject should probably go untreated. In other circumstances, VT is a life-threatening arrhythmia and demands prompt conversion. Treatment is particularly urgent in acute myocardial infarction, hypokalemia, and digitalis intoxication.

In <u>acute myocardial infarction</u>, VT of recent onset usually responds to low energy countershock (10-20 joules); if the patient is stable, it is reasonable to try a bolus of lidocaine, but if this fails to convert the arrhythmia promptly, no time should be lost in terminating the VT electrically. Note that in the presence of significant hypotension, no antiarrhythmic measure may be effective until the blood pressure has been artificially jacked up.

In <u>hypokalemia</u>, potassium is clearly the agent of choice. In <u>digitalis intoxication</u>, countershcok is to be avoided and the most important measure is discontinuation of the drug; potassium may be useful, and among the antiarrhythmic agents, propranolol, phenytoin, and perhaps lidocaine, may prove effective.

To prevent recurrences in the acute situation, a continuous lidocaine or procainamide drip is effective. For prolonged prevention, propranolol, mexiletine, disopyramide, quinidine, moricizine or propafenone may all be tried; in desperation, one may turn to amiodarone. The drug selected is more likely to be effective if one is guided by electrophysiological studies. The combination of a beta-blocker with a IA or IB agent may be more effective than any single preparation. In view of the CAST experience, it is best to avoid the IC agents (flecainide, encainide).

GENERAL APPROACH TO TREATMENT OF SUPRAVENTRICULAR TACHYCARDIAS

<u>Sinus tachycardia</u> is usually compensatory and requires palliation or removal of cause, eg, heart failure, hypoxia, etc. If temporary slowing seems worth while, I-V esmolol may be effective for a few minutes, or propranolol for a longer period.

<u>A-V nodal reentrant tachycardia</u> is usually not urgent, often occuring in healthy hearts. Simple measures first: rest, sedation, vagal stimulation. If further intervention needed, digoxin, varapamil (or diltiazem), or propranolol (or other beta blocker) are all effective. For most rapid response, adenosine in I-V bolus.

If above are ineffective and situation is urgent because of associated heart disease, DC cardioversion or right atrial pacing may be needed.

For prevention of attacks, oral digitalis, quinidine, propranolol, or verapamil may be effective. Ablation or surgical procedures very rarely needed.

<u>Reentrant tachycardia using an accessory pathway</u>. Because of the everpresent risk that atrial flutter or fibrillation may develop, drugs that facilitate accessory pathway conduction (digoxin, verapamil, lidocaine) are best avoided.

Vagal stimulation may be tried. Propranolol and class I drugs (quinidine, procainamide, disopyramide) are often effective. If not, DC cardioversion.

To prevent recurrences, amiodarone is very effective but seldom advocated because of inordinate incidence and seriousness of side-effects. Severely symptomatic patients should have electrophysiological studies followed by pathway ablation or surgery.

<u>Ectopic atrial tachycardia</u>. Although learned texts often describe this as a persistent tachycardia, short, self-terminating bursts are quite common in the real world. Usually secondary to a significant abnormality, it is often unresponsive to antiarrhythmic agents and only responds to palliation or removal of the underlying cause, eg, heart failure, myocardial ischemia, hypoxia, digitalis intoxication, electrolyte imbalance, etc.

Paroxysms may be—but usually are not—reduced or prevented by drugs such as digoxin, quinidine, propranolol, verapamil or moricizine.

In <u>multifocal atrial tachycardia</u>, most often associated with chronic lung disease, verapamil or diltiazem may be effective; propranolol should be avoided, and most other drugs are ineffective.

109

NOTE: If QRS is wide, and ventricular tachycardia is mistaken for supraventricular with aberration, verapamil can cause hypotension, shock and/or ventricular fibrillation; therefore, unless absolutely sure of the diagnosis, one should avoid verapamil when treating wide-QRS tachycardias.

GENERAL APPROACH TO TREATMENT OF ATRIAL FLUTTER

As with atrial fibrillation, one should always keep two goals in mind: Controlling the ventricular rate, and converting the arrhythmia to restore a normal atrial kick. Sometimes one goal is predominant, sometimes the other.

Atrial flutter occurs almost exclusively in diseased hearts, though it may be precipitated by extracardiac catastrophes. The arrhythmia is sensitive to DC counter-shock, usually responding to low dosage (10-50 joules); therefore, if the ventricular rate is dangerously rapid, the attending physician must decide whether to employ electrical conversion promptly, or to slow the ventricular rate by increasing A-V block with I-V digoxin, propranolol or verapamil—the choice much depends upon his evaluation of the relative urgency of the situation. Because of the possiblity that countershock may still be required, one may prefer to use one of the other two drugs rather than digoxin; and in the presence of known or suspected accessory pathways, both digoxin and verapamil should be avoided. If the rate is successfully slowed by I-V medication, the improved perfusion may itself correct the arrhythmia.

If the ventricular rate is controlled but the flutter persists, conversion may be achieved with countershock, or with drugs, of which quinidine is usually first choice, though both procainamide and disopyramide may succeed.

If the ventricular rate is controlled but the flutter persists, conversion can be ap-proached either electrically or pharmacologically. Since quinidine favors A-V con-duction and may therefore accelerate the ventricular response, it should be administered only after digitalization.

To prevent recurrences, a combination of quinidine and digoxin is generally used; the class IC agents (flecainide, encainide) may also be effective. Very rarely, surgical or ablative procedures must be resorted to.

GENERAL APPROACH TO TREATMENT OF ATRIAL FIBRILLATION

Always keep two goals in mind:

   1) Control the ventricular rate, and

   2) Restore atrial kick by converting to sinus rhythm.

At times one goal is uppermost, at times the other.

Be sure to seek and cope with underlying pathology (if any), such as hypertension, thyrotoxicosis, rheumatic (especially mitral) disease, myocardial ischemia, pulmonary emboli, atrial septal defect, pericarditis, etc. Also remember that heart failure may be the cause of atrial fibrillation, and atrial fibrillation may be the cause of heart failure.

Paroxysmal:

   a) to prevent recurrences: digoxin + quinidine (simultaneous administration of digoxin important to control ventricular rate which quinidine may accelerate), class IC agents (flecainide, encainide). If heart failure is the underlying cause of the fibrillation, digoxin alone may suffice.

   b) to terminate paroxysm: quinidine (under digitalis umbrella), or DC cardioversion.

Persistent: Control rate with digoxin, propranolol or verapamil; then convert with quinidine or DC cardioversion.

Chronic: Control ventricular rate (as above).

Cardioversion may be attempted—lasting success unlikely.

Anticoagulation is controversial—it may offer some protection against embolism but carries intrinsic risks.

GENERAL APPROACH TO TREATMENT OF SICK SINUS SYNDROMES

The ailing sinus node manifests its discomfiture in several ways: marked sinus bradycardia (enabling subsidiary pacemakers to escape with consequent various bradyarrhythmic patterns—such as #43); sinus pauses or arrest; various bradycardia-tachycardia combinations; etc. Some patients with demonstrably sick sinuses have no symptoms, and there is no evidence that pacemaker therapy prolongs life; it should therefore be reserved for patients who are symptomatic; in them the quality of life is improved and the risk of accidental death diminished.

The acute sick sinus, as manifested, for example, by sinus bradycardia in acute inferior infarction, can often be satisfactorily controlled with judicious dosage of I-V atropine; isoproterenol is effective, but has the disadvantage of increasing the oxygen requirement of the myocardium. An external, temporary pacemaker may occasionally be needed.

Treatment of the chronic sick sinus is simple, since there is only one effective mode, the artificial pacemaker—and the sick sinus has become the most common indication for implantation. As long as A-V block complicates a significant number of sick sinus syndromes, it may be prophylactically wise to install a dual chamber model programmed in the AAI mode.

GENERAL APPROACH TO TREATMENT OF A-V BLOCK

The two most important considerations in assessing the seriousness of A-V block are (1) the resulting VENTRICULAR rate and (2) the anatomical level of the block. By and large, if the ventricular rate is adequate and the block is A-V nodal, no treatment is necessary; but if the block is infranodal, regardless of the ventricular rate, it is bad news, forebodes worse trouble, and demands intervention by pacing.

In acute A-V nodal block, as with inferior infarction, usually no treatment is necessary. Sometimes the ventricular rate is inadequate and I-V atropine improves the conduction ratio; isoproterenol also is effective, but significantly increases the oxygen requirement of the myocardium and is better avoided. Rarely a temporary external pacemaker may be necessary to maintain the ventricular rate at an acceptable level. If genuine complete block (ventricular rate under 45/min) develops acutely, a temporary pacemaker is clearly indicated.

If type II A-V block develops acutely, as with an anteroseptal infarction, a temporary pacemaker is indicated immediately, regardless of the ventricular rate.

Any unequivocal manifestation of chronic type II block and chronic complete A-V block with a ventricular rate under 45/min are indications for a permanent pacemaker. The form of pacemaker installed depends on the patient's age, life-style, etc.

Also available

POCKET PROFESSOR SETS

Five sets of laminated cards containing valuable "fingertip" information.
About Twelve - 3" x 4 1/2" laminated cards with hinged ring.

CCU Pocket Professor (2nd ed.)
by Jonni Cooper, RN
- Includes arrhythmias, blocks, drug therapies
- Ventricular ectopy/aberration, bundle branch block, hemiblock
- Axis quadrants, axis in degrees
- Atrioventricular block, myocardial infarction patterns
- Normal 12-Lead placement, intravenous drug equivalents
- Antiarrhythmic agents/dosages, arrhythmias & therapies
- Antianginal agents/dosages, angina patterns

ICU Pocket Professor (2nd ed.)
by Jonni Cooper, RN
- Includes physical signs, symptoms, lab data
- Hemodynamic monitoring facts, figures, problem solving
- History taking, physical assessment of the CV system
- Heart and lung sounds, lung conditions
- Calculating blood gases I and II
- Cardiac enzymes, normal lab values

Antiarrhythmic Pocket Professor (2nd ed.)
by Henry J.L. Marriott, MD, FACP, FACC
- Antiarrhythmic drugs by class, when to use antiarrhythmics
- Quinidine, Procainamide, Disopyramide, Lidocaine
- Tocainide, Phenytoin, Mexiletine, Flecainide
- Propafenone, Propranolol, Esmolol, Digoxin
- Bretylium, Amiodarone, Verapamil, Adenosine, Moricizine

Pacemakers Pocket Professor (2nd ed.)
by Jonni Cooper, RN
- The revised five-position ICHD code
- General indications for pacemaker implantation
- Pacemaker definitions, complications of implants
- Ventricular demand (VVI), VVI pacing
- Atrial demand (AAI), AAI pacing
- AV sequential (DVI), DVI pacing
- VDD pacing, DDD (Automatic), DDD pacing

Life-Threatening Arrhythmias/Therapy Pocket Professor
by Jonni Cooper, RN
- Ventricular fibrillation (VF), tachycardia (VT)
- Morphologic features of arrhythmias
- Comparing ventricular ectopy with aberrant conduction
- Idioventricular rhythm, accelerated idioventricular rhythm
- Agonal rhythm, asystole
- Electrical mechanical dissociation (EMD)
- Torsades de pointes
- Determining an electrical axis, determining axis in exact degrees
- Atrial fibrillation (AF), flutter and many more